THE A.R.T. OF

Dental Healing

A theater of discovery for reclaiming your excellent healthy teeth!

ROBERT GODBOUT

Cover by Marianny R – @mrnny_art

Interior Design & Formatting by Andrea Iturra

Contributor: Arpita Paul – literatureabbey.com

Consultant: Fatuma

To the Holy Ones

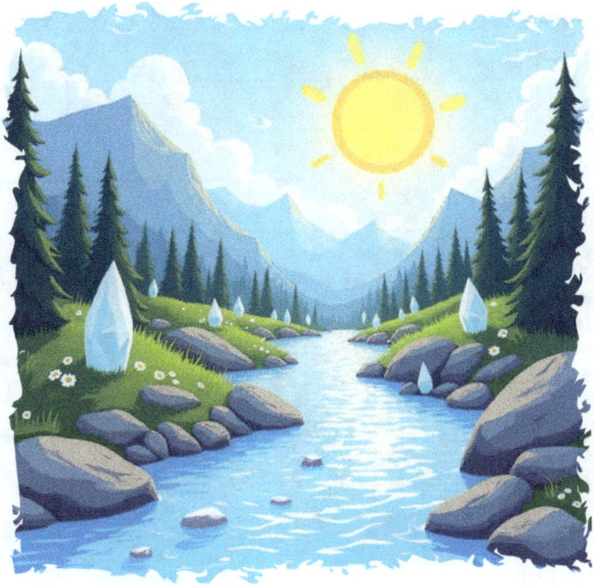

Table of Contents

Disclaimer

The information contained in this text is provided for educational and informational purposes only. It is not intended as a substitute for professional medical advice, diagnosis, or treatment from a qualified healer (dentist or healthcare provider).

No Doctor-Patient Relationship: Reading or using this information does not establish a doctor-patient relationship between you and the author.

Not Medical Advice: The author is not a licensed medical professional. The content, including any text, graphics, images, or other material, is for general informational purposes and represents the author's personal research and opinions. It should not be solely depended upon for wellness-related decisions.

Individual Results Vary: Every individual's health and healing process is unique. The outcomes, results, and healing timelines mentioned are anecdotal and may not be typical. You should not expect to achieve any predetermined result.

Consult Your Healing Professional: Always seek the advice of your healer (a dentist or another qualified health provider) with any questions you may have regarding a dental or medical condition. Never disregard professional medical advice or delay seeking it because of something you have read in this text.

No Endorsements: Mention of any specific product, procedure, or service does not constitute an endorsement or recommendation by the author.

Assumption of Risk: You assume all risk for any actions you take or refrain from taking based on the content of this text. The author shall not be held liable or responsible for any loss, injury, or damage allegedly arising from any information or suggestion contained herein.

1 CHAPTER

Hard *Reckoning*

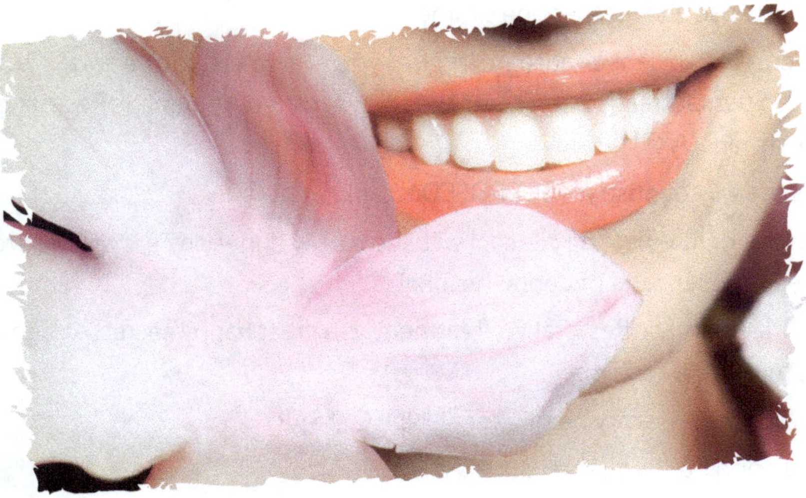

Core points:

1. Dentistry must be enjoyable, not scary.
2. It also becomes healthier.
3. Wellness relates to abundance.
4. Industrial dentistry is the wrong path.

Dentistry was never supposed to be scary and painful! It was always meant to be enjoyable, relaxing, yes, even fun.

This is correct dentistry.

Why is dentistry so toxic? The materials, the methods.

Let's be clear: dentistry gives you a business experience rather than a healing experience!

Let's pause and let that one simmer.

There is an ancient dentistry that gives you everything you've always wanted in dental treatment. This ancient way is called Atraumatic Restorative Treatment (ART).

It's the way dentistry is SUPPOSED to be!

I'm the dental healing coach. I will show how unhealthy dentistry becomes a golden land of dental healing!

ART (Atraumatic Restorative Treatment) is a great happy secret! Atraumatic means, NO trauma.

In most cases, scary needles are UNNECESSARY!

They don't tell you that! But it's true!

In most cases, scary mechanical drilling is wrong, and completely unnecessary!

They don't tell you that either!

Yes, this is all shocking! Are we having fun yet?

Let's make a list. Lists are fun.

1. We want healthy teeth to last a lifetime.
2. We need a MAGIC BOOK to show us how!
3. Hopefully, it's written by the Tooth Fairy, or one of her close associates.
4. Where's that Magic Book? We have an appointment coming soon!

Some may argue: Are you saying that ALL dental treatments are going to be enjoyable and painless?

Truth is, MOST will be. The only exceptions are the few emergency treatments that require the "surgery" that dentistry does on a regular basis!

ART is your new best friend! (Chapter 14 explains the essence of the protocol.)

Happy dentistry is the win-win situation!

The difference between regular dentistry and correct, happy dentistry is massive.

Traditional dentistry now has a name: "Rockefeller dentistry".

This name is not patented and you are free to use it often!

100 years ago there was a rapid shift to industrialization. Heavy industry, but also education, medicine, and ....dentistry!

Industrialization and mass production was fine for manufacturing. The problem is: Teeth are not machinery!

Dentistry was separated from medicine. No longer part of medical insurance disbursements and billing cycles.

Doctors couldn't check oral health anymore. Dentists could no longer examine your ankles.

The human body remains ONE integral unit! (Notably on weekends and statutory holidays.)

You DO NOT want a doctor using a high-speed dental bur on your rear end. But neither do you want a dentist doing surgery every time you visit. Yet he works in an operatory!

People are terrified of dentistry!

WHY?

It has to come back from the abyss.

We need famous people to regale us with their knowledge, their secrets. Their clever one-liners!

Otherwise, kaput! The time is short. We need answers!

Mikhail sure knows it...

2
CHAPTER

Chekhov 1

Stepping back in time, where the good doctor CHEKHOV met dentistry!

Title: The Reluctant Driller-Dentist

Scene: A modest dental office in a provincial Russian town, late 19th century.

The walls are lined with ominous-looking instruments. A large, antiquated drill sits in the corner, its foot pedal worn from use.

Ivan Petrovich, a weary dentist with a perpetually resigned expression, stands over his tray of tools, sighing.

Enter Mikhail Sergeyevich, a nervous but determined gentleman in a slightly frayed suit.

Mikhail Sergeyevich: (*removing his hat and wringing it in his hands*)
"Ivan Petrovich, good day. I've come about my teeth."

Ivan Petrovich: (*without looking up*)
"Ah. Which ones?"

Mikhail Sergeyevich: (*pointing gingerly to his cheek*)
"All of them, in fact…"

Ivan Petrovich: (*nods, reaching for a probe*)
"Then we shall drill."

Mikhail Sergeyevich: (*flinching*)
"No! No drilling. Only ART atraumatic restorative treatment."

Ivan Petrovich: (*pausing, squinting*)
"…What?"

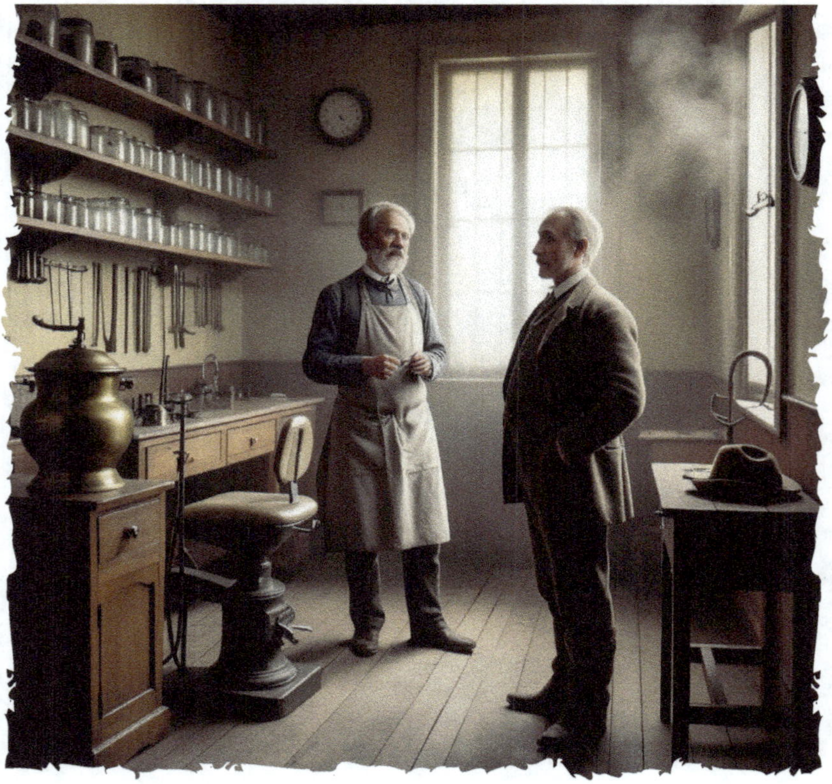

Mikhail Sergeyevich: (*leaning in, earnest*)
"It's the modern approach, but in fact, also the most ancient. No drills, no pain - just a small spoon, some glass ionomer, and patience. It's ten times more healthy!"

Ivan Petrovich: (*laughs darkly, gesturing to the drill*)
"Healthier? My friend, this drill has served me for 20 years. It sings like a samovar at full boil. Why dig with a teaspoon when you have a proper shovel?"

Mikhail Sergeyevich:
"But... the trauma..."

Ivan Petrovich: (*cutting him off, wistful*)
"Life is trauma, Mikhail Sergeyevich.
The tooth decays. The drill turns. We suffer, and then... we drink tea."

Mikhail Sergeyevich:
"There is a dental healer. His name is Vasily. His methods are minimally invasive. He saves teeth."

Ivan Petrovich: (*shrugging, picking up his forceps*)
"Then you may keep your teeth… until they rot entirely, and we must pull them like bad potatoes. Or, crowns and implants of course. (*sighs.*) But suit yourself."
(*A long pause. The clock ticks. Mikhail stares at the drill, then at the ceiling.*)

Mikhail Sergeyevich:
"He saves teeth, Ivan Petrovich."

Ivan Petrovich:
"Yes, you mentioned it."

Mikhail Sergeyevich:
"A sapling bends before the winter winds. It lives to see the spring. Many springs. Does your drill really sing?"

Ivan Petrovich:
"Like a lark, my friend. Like a lark."

Mikhail Sergeyevich:
"Vasily has a solution, Ivan Petrovich. It dissolves the decay. It prevents loss. Resisting change requires a different type of solution, however. A solution yes, but different."

Ivan Petrovich:
"Sergeyevar Sergeyevich, the drill is all we know!"
Mikhail Sergeyevich:
"Then surely we know little. Excuse me. I need to consider."

Ivan Petrovich:
"Then, please do. And let me know."

Mikhail Sergeyevich:
"I shall, Ivan Petrovich."
(*Fadeout.*)

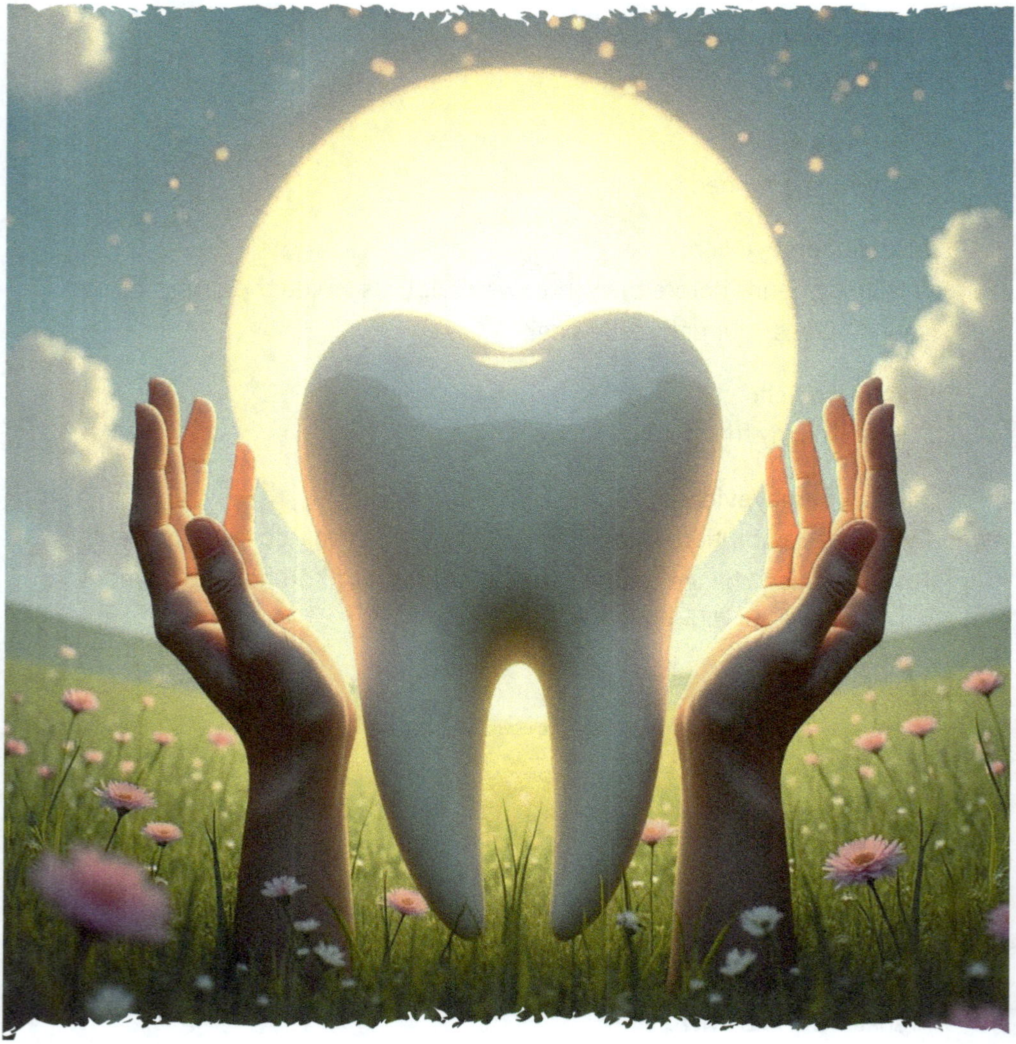

3

CHAPTER

Objectives

Core points:

1. Healthier, plus more enjoyable, work together well.
2. The ultra-basics of good oral health.
3. Dentists often don't know what's best or healthiest.
4. Drilling and pain control are in the majority of cases not needed.
5. A healthier method that's also pain-free is a fabulous win-win.

Good dental health comes with a price. And that price is… happiness! Did you see that loop coming?

To have great dental health means that you're going to have to give up all your pain and suffering!

It's almost illogical!

Are we ready for it?

Our dental healing journey is our ladder to truth. The dental industry is a business. They know it, we know it.

We're not here to apologize for this huge business! We're here to heal dentally!

Will we do it? Of course!

We start with some super-basics for excellent dental health. These are the foundation:

1. **Smart Oral Hygiene.** Brushing and flossing often (especially after any processed food) to remove plaque and food in crevices, and using an excellent dentifrice. Chapter 56 is about making your own toothpaste!

2. **Diet & Sugar Control.** Eliminate all sugary and acidic foods (e.g. soda, candy) that erode enamel. Eat calcium-rich foods (dairy, leafy greens) for strong teeth. An alkaline oral pH is super beneficial.
3. **Dental Checkups with Healers Only.** No more injurious dentistry. Cleanings by healing hygienists will remove tartar buildup.
4. **Accepting the Abundance of Dental Longevity.** Your teeth are designed to last as long as your body. Taking total control of your dental health journey is so important.
5. **Avoiding Harmful Dentistry** (Yes, this is a key factor!) Poor fillings, crowns, or most drilling will greatly weaken your teeth. Do choose minimally invasive dentistry every time. Choose ART, the Gold Standard.

These basics are sure to bring good results. Number five is the wildcard here. It's the one we need to discuss in depth.

If we're going to heal dentally we have to go straight to the solution!

Frank Jerome, a fashionably rogue dentist, said that up to 90% of dental treatment diagnoses are entirely optional and negotiable. An amazing confession from a low-handicap dentist!

(Frank broke down after making that statement, but he was soon well again.)

Most people automatically trust what their dentist tells them. (Not me, but others). That's because he has a white lab coat and a four-plus years degree on the wall! He looks the part!

If it looks like a dentist, it must be a dentist! If it looks like Ivan Petrovich, it must be Ivan Petrovich!

The dentist has a high overhead (big office and staff) and a tight schedule. He can't be missing tee times! The big power tools are there to make the job quicker.

Not safer or healthier, mind you. Just quicker. Less chair time. And the reception is often in on the sale!

Do any of those tools and procedures work for the health and longevity of your teeth? Now we're asking the dangerous questions. Dental longevity talk!

Nearly all modern dentistry is not even close to what it's supposed to be. A real coach kicks serious butt, and I'm here to do just that.

Is it fake, then? Fake is a tough term. How about, does it serve itself more than it serves you? Ah, now we're getting somewhere!

In essence, we could say that after our findings, dentistry as we currently know it should start to dissolve, break up, and crumble.

And in its place shall grow a new dentistry, one that serves YOU before it serves itself!

Now that's nailing it! (Appropriate coaches bark.)

When you get a dental procedure, you intend to get healthier, not to be injured.

However, every time a dental high-speed drill is applied to your living teeth, the lifespan of those teeth shortens. Sometimes by a lot.

In other words, it gets injured!

Many high-quality studies prove beyond a doubt that high-speed drills are very injurious to the delicate structure of the teeth.

Wait! Is this to say that nearly all dentists, 99% of them in developed countries, are purposely injuring you?

Not intentionally. What it proves is that the "needle and drill" method is definitely injurious, and that, at the very core of things, it is completely UNNECESSARY.

This outrageousness has a powerful substrate of logic to it. Logic plus passion! Enough with pretending!

And what are the alternatives to this "injurious dentistry", you're probably asking.

Here's the HAPPY reality: the alternatives to painful, stressful, traumatic dentistry, are...

Enjoyable!

Relaxing!

Stress-free!

Plus....

MUCH healthier!

Can this be possible? Can something that's much better for you, something much healthier.... also be more enjoyable?

(Time for a magical pause.)

Yes, THAT is the elegant solution!

So THIS is the high abundance we hear about! This is the VERY good stuff!

It's how good leads to good. It's where the real magic begins.

Yes, it's almost inconceivable. But that's because people are far too often expecting bad, painful dentistry. And when good healing dentistry finally arrives, there's euphoria!

There are at least a dozen excellent research studies that might well knock your socks off! Easier when you're wearing sandals!

They all prove the injurious nature of the current mainstream dentistry. Are we ready for some serious smack-talk?

Summary: Modern dentistry is in the majority of cases injurious, but there is a 100% healing dentistry called ART.

Being the ancient way, it's also the most healing.

Don't vilify the dentist, but instead the very inappropriate business-based education he got. That's the focus. We're here to heal!

And to outline the process, we drop into a Greek olive grove where a scintillating meeting is taking place! Oh my goodness. we've seen these names before....

4

CHAPTER

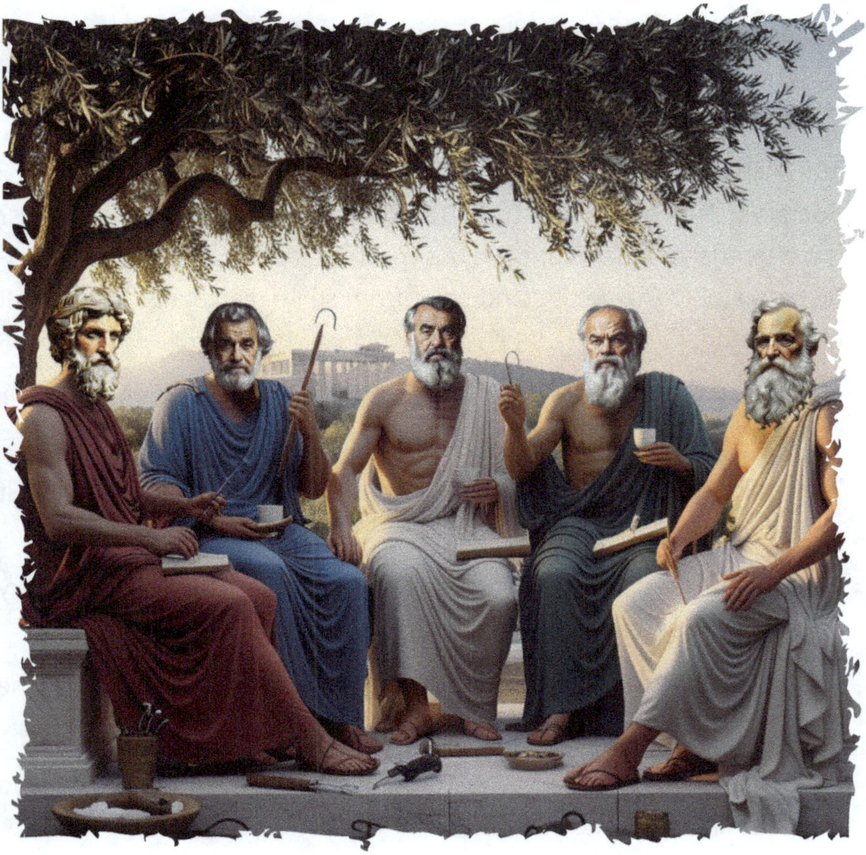

Dentagora

Title: The Five Dental Philosophers

Setting: A shaded grove near the Athenian agora, where five illustrious philosophers gather under the olive trees as the sun sets, casting long shadows.

1. Socrates (*The questioning dentist*)
2. Plato (*The idealist dentist*)
3. Aristotle (*The empirical endodontist*)
4. Parmenides (*The Minimally Invasive mystic*)
5. Heraclitus (*The obscure hygienist*)

The Dialogue:

Socrates: "Friends, we seek truth. Yet what is it? Is it in us? Is it outside us? Is it over there, under that olive bush? Is truth apprehensible in the dental marketplace? Does it stand apart from smile marketing? How about on weekends?"

Heraclitus: "Truth is a flame. It blazes. It morphs. We learn from nature. Financially, no need to fear. Our industry is so profitable."

Parmenides: "But it sits on the precipice of change. It's not sustainable. It doesn't heal!"

Plato: "The wisest of us admits that he knows little. About real dentistry anyway. The new cafe down the road does cinnamon lattes."

Aristotle: "The ideal of excellence must prevail! Asclepios said that the Light reveals the essence."

Parmenides: "The light! Gateway of Mithra. But more. We comprehend Buddhist dharma. History forgot."

Aristotle: "Secrets of time."

Socrates: "Our kind drills, fills, and bills. Did we forget the basic premise of our craft?"

Aristotle: "The premise to heal and not to injure? Excellence becomes a habit. Regrettably, so does its opposite."

Plato: "Dental excellence. Form, not shadow."

Heraclitus: "An ideal dentistry?"

Plato: "There is, there is."

Parmenides: "The minimally invasive healing method alone describes truth. It also transcends obsession with chair time."

Socrates: "The search for ideal dentistry is that Light."

Plato: "Enough with billing cycles and chair time."

Heraclitus: "I keep short hours. My golf scores are pretty good."

Aristotle: "Drilling trauma is needless."

Parmenides: "Naming the thing helps us to recognize its nature. Hermione said that in front of Lucius."

Heraclitus: "Audacity."

Socrates: "We need solutions."

Plato: "Solutions are there when the lazy use of the drill is tossed."

Aristotle: "Obvious."

The group settles back and refills their glasses with fragrant retsina. The Sun dips below the horizon, casting an iridescent glow on the landscape and rendering the men's forms akin to fire.

Socrates: (glancing at Parmenides) "There is a marvel, friends: a healer who removes decay not violently but by alliance with the tooth's own form."

Parmenides: "I resemble that allegation."

Plato: "The ideal form! The excellence of craft!"

Aristotle: "Courage also. Four years of stinking science-based curriculum. Cynical industrial habit patterns."

Heraclitus: "Trauma-free! Wellness proves the truth. True craft."

Parmenides: "Speaking of what exists…"

Plato: "How could this training obscure that ideal form?"

Aristotle: "Ah, the curriculum. Did it become a greed funnel?"

Heraclitus: "Damned greed!"

Socrates: "Our training sucked."

Plato: "Dentists, we're not absolved of poor quality because we gazed at shadows. Our six figures obsession got in the way."

Heraclitus: "My success bootcamp disagrees with this."

Parmenides: "True dentistry. There is always such a thing."

Plato: "I shall examine my craft again."

Socrates: "The true dentistry is…"

Parmenides: "Essentially painless, plus healthier. Two for one."

Aristotle: "Efaristo, bro!"

Plato: "Symfonos!"

Socrates: "A metaphor for wisdom itself!"

Heraclitus: "To a terrified client, much more than metaphor."

Parmenides: "I rejected half of that curriculum."

Socrates: "Let me be your student then."

Plato: "Sincerity is our best teacher."

Aristotle: "Reconditioning on a large scale?"

Socrates: "One step at a time."

Parmenides: "Brother Plato, why don't the people rebel against these frightening methods?"

Plato: "Unaware of a true way."

Heraclitus: "The atraumatic way shall be the best thing that's happened to them."

Aristotle: "They need to know…"

Plato: "Dentists need to know…"

Aristotle: "To heal, not to overtreat. To comprehend dental longevity."

Socrates: "Truer than billing cycles!"

Parmenides: "Our little agora, in this apricot grove!"

Socrates: "Truly, brother."

Parmenides: "Truly so."

Heraclitus: "Hear. Refill my cup!"

5

CHAPTER

Reality Check

Core points:

1. Serious studies have proven that drilling teeth causes injury.
2. Dental education often contains false assumptions.
3. The curriculum does not emphasize long-term health.
4. It focuses on expensive repair.
5. Dental students are taught harmful practices.
6. Longevity is not a guiding principle of the dental college curriculum.

Let's make some very bold claims. Yes! Right here, right now:

1. Modern dentistry routinely injures you.
2. There is an ancient healing dentistry called ART.
3. Modern dentistry hasn't adopted it (YET) because it's not as profitable as the usual invasive, injurious dentistry.

Yes, these are outrageous claims, yet they do stand up nicely. Dentistry is not supposed to injure you when you go to have treatment for a restoration. Not one bit!

The top five studies describing the whole thing were done by:

1. Banerjee
2. Brännström
3. Elderton

4. Periera
5. Fusayama

The essence of these studies (and many other similar high-quality ones) is that the heat and vibration of drilling weakens tooth structure, causes micro-fractures and pulp trauma, and leads to premature loss of teeth.

Let's ponder this for a moment. Hard stuff!

Everyone who's even been for a dental treatment knows the experience all too well.

So is the above claim provable? Hold on! This is where it gets real good!

Modern dentistry is a very "closed-shop" industry where barriers to entry are very high and expensive.

But does actual healing take place here? That's always the first question to ask.

"Dental cavity" is how dentistry describes the work environment. Most interesting because it's obviously a passage for the flow of air, food, and nervous impulse. And even things we know less about. Like, a passage for laughing.

Dentistry calls it a cavity. Wrong! It is not a big "gravel pit" to play with your toys in!

In the dental college third-year Endodontics course (where they teach recruits how to kill a tooth and place latex inside it), the diagram they use shows a very smooth dentinal wall.

It doesn't show the thousands of microtubules there, the vessel pockets which carry the blood to the pulp. These will potentially harbor harmful bacteria.

The instructor just goes "Hey! Let's just pretend it's not there!"

Dental college doesn't seem to know or care much what Ozone is.

With a 99.9% success rate for eliminating harmful bacteria, and enabling rapid healing of tissue, they're probably just terrified of it.

Of course they are! It works so well and has no harmful side effects!

Is dental college a "ship of fools"? They sure seem to be trying.

These colleges are high security installations. They don't want anyone dropping in to suggest safer, healthier courses.

There have been serious, egregious deceptions in the history of dentistry. As in, mercury fillings.

Millions have been injured by these "amalgams" because mercury is such a toxic neuropoison. These fillings contain up to 50% concentrations of mercury.

Besides being extremely poisonous, the procedure requires the removal of healthy tissue for anchoring, which is iatrogenic in the extreme.

Many people have needed to remove all these mercury amalgam fillings at their own cost because the dental profession will never admit to needing to fix the mistake they made. And all these fillings need to be replaced to prevent continued poisoning.

It's very scandalous! In an ideally ethical situation, dentistry would readily reimburse clients for the harms they have actually caused!

From personal experience, removing mercury amalgam fillings is like having a big weight lifted off the shoulders. The relief is immense.

One reason why it's hard to forget about it is that it's still in the dental college curriculum. Incredible but true. And it's also being used in some pediatric dentistry.

Mercury is the second most poisonous substance after plutonium.

Dental industry: "Oops, you called us out on it. Okay, nothing to see here, folks. Move along now." What an abysmal attitude!

Dentistry needs to be enjoyable, relaxing, and stress-free, as well as very healthy. It isn't, though!

Frank Jerome says that the majority of dental treatments are to repair or treat previously done treatments. It's a revolving wheel! Not a good prospect for dental longevity.

And it starts and ends with the dental college curriculum. This is where the buck stops.

The unfortunate outcome of bad and invasive dentistry is that many people assume that their teeth are destined to eventually fall out and be replaced with artificial ones.

This resignation is very wrong. Teeth are meant to last as long as you do.

DENTAL LONGEVITY is the way. Dental healing is a HIGH adventure, and rewarding on all levels.

I came full circle in my comprehension of dentistry. Things will never be the same!

I will describe this in the context of a small Mexican village for dental expats! I now have full confidence in what works and what doesn't in dentistry.

This journey is presented in the form of serious subject matter alternating with parody. We must laugh!

So let's get on with it. It's a heck of a ride! Let's strap in!

6

CHAPTER

Evidence 1

Core points:

1. Drilling teeth is a very misguided habit.
2. A Pereira study proved that microfractures result from drilling.
3. A Frencken study proved that hand-instrument treatments are vastly superior.
4. Zach and Cohen proved that heat from drilling causes deep tooth trauma.
5. Why do dentists insist on drilling?
6. The dental college curriculum requires serious reconsideration.

"I'm sorry, but we have to use a drill. There's no other choice."

"And a needle injection?"

"Of course. We don't want you jumping around in the chair."

Regrettably, this is a familiar dental clinic conversation. What if you'll never have to hear this again? Ever!

Too good to be true? Hold on. The tooth fairy has great news for you!

Those great studies done on the harm caused by dental drills seems to be mostly unknown to the public. And, it's for all too obvious reasons.

For one, the industry makes a ton of money from expensive treatments. And two, they like it when you keep coming back!

Am I being dangerous yet? Let me know and I'll pause 30 seconds before I continue!

Seriously, we need to be disruptive here, because there is so much deception to disrupt!

A timeless quote goes: "The more you treat the teeth with invasive mechanical instruments (and believe me, nearly everything in dentistry is invasive), the weaker the teeth become."

Now that quote is catchy!

Let's get to the studies!

Brazilian dentist Dr. Cláudio Pereira was instrumental in the early research and promotion of ART alongside Dutchman Jo Frencken.

His 2015 study was published in the *Journal of the Mechanical Behavior of Biomedical Materials*. The study compared the effects of high-speed (300,000+ rpm) vs. low-speed (40,000 rpm) dental drills.

The key outcomes of the study were as follows:

1. Microcracks up to a depth of 300 microns occur with high-speed drills, which is 10% of the total dentin thickness).
2. The drills result in "sonic fatigue" in the dentin's collagen matrix.
3. Microfractures radiate outward from the drill site (like a windshield crack).
4. Low-speed drills were slightly less but with torque-induced cracks from burs "grabbing" dentin.
5. Restoration bond strength was weakened, with marginal leakage.

A 2018 study by Yaman confirmed these findings. The micro-cracks exposed fluid-filled dentin tubules.

A Bajaj follow-up study confirmed that at least 60% of drilled teeth show microcracks:

1. If non-symptomatic, they still accelerate tooth aging.
2. Drills often inadvertently remove healthy tooth structure.

A follow-up study by Frencken showed that ART treatment results in zero high-frequency vibration and no sonic fatigue:

1. ART results in no torque cracks.
2. Teeth treated with ART show 90% fewer microcracks vs. drilled teeth.
3. The dentists continue to use drills because they are 3x to 5x faster than ART.
4. Insurance-based practices profit from the time savings.

Pereira said: "Microcracks are the hidden cost of 'efficient' drilling. We trade minutes in the chair for years of tooth lifespan."

Put this quote on your wall! Make it a mantra before your next dental appointment.

Zach and Cohen in 1965 studied heat damage from drills. Their study revealed:

1. Temperatures above 55°C cause irreversible pulp necrosis in a large percentage of teeth.
2. Water-cooling doesn't instantly penetrate to the cutting interface where heat is generated. Microseconds of heat exposure still occur.
3. Poor spray alignment or clogged ports lead to dry zones where heat builds unchecked.
4. Many teeth suffer subclinical pulp inflammation after drilling, leading to premature aging of the tooth and a delayed need for root canals
5. Atraumatic methods (hand tools, chemomechanical caries removal) result in zero heat damage.

A Banerjee study in 2000 confirmed earlier studies on subsurface cracks. Hand excavation with ART was proven to preserve over 95% more healthy tissue.

A 1982 Endod study confirmed that the mechanical trauma plus heat during drilling triggers pulp inflammation, resulting in frequent root canals.

A Mickenautsch study in 2007 showed that ART restorations have superior longevity to drill fillings, with better seal quality.

A Souza (Brazil) 2021 study on thousands of clients showed an above 90% 10-year restoration survival rate for ART treatment compared to under 40% for drill treatments. The ART restorations averaged 80% less follow-up care over a decade.

Many of these studies grew out of the 1965 study by Brännström, which will be discussed in Chapter 52 of this volume.
[These high quality studies and several others are citation-referenced in the rear pages of this volume.]

There is some serious disruption here. These findings demolish the entire rationale for using a high-speed drill.

We have to wonder why the dental industry hasn't taken this evidence and made the necessary corrections.

Now you know why it's "Rockefeller dentistry". Does it serve YOU, or does it serve itself?

These studies did have some positive effects however. They laid the foundation for the following:

- Minimally invasive dentistry (MID).
- Biomimetic restorative techniques.
- Modern caries removal systems (e.g., lasers, Carisolv).

In other words, they woke a lot of people up and had them devise ways to make dentistry safer.

So the question remains: Why do nearly all dentists choose drilling as the only option? It comes down to:

- Speed/convenience of burs.

- Lack of training in alternatives.

- Profit models favoring drill-based procedures.

There's tremendous inertia, and a lot of it is with the dental college curriculum. Despite these scorching studies, the basic curriculum didn't really change at all.

I've investigated that curriculum. It's four years of serious and hard science! But it also appears to be a business education.

When your teeth are great, fit, and healthy, you don't have to return for a lot more treatment. It's good news for you, but maybe not for them!

Do you really want to keep subsidizing expensive dentistry as your teeth gradually become extinct?

Every needle injection and drilling experience shortens the lifespan of a tooth. These studies prove it. And there are many more highly reputable studies that echo these.

How about a new happy declaration: "I will never allow a high-speed drill into my oral passage (not a cavity!) ever again.

That's the START OF ART. A new day dawns. But for Elizabethan England, it took a mighty struggle...

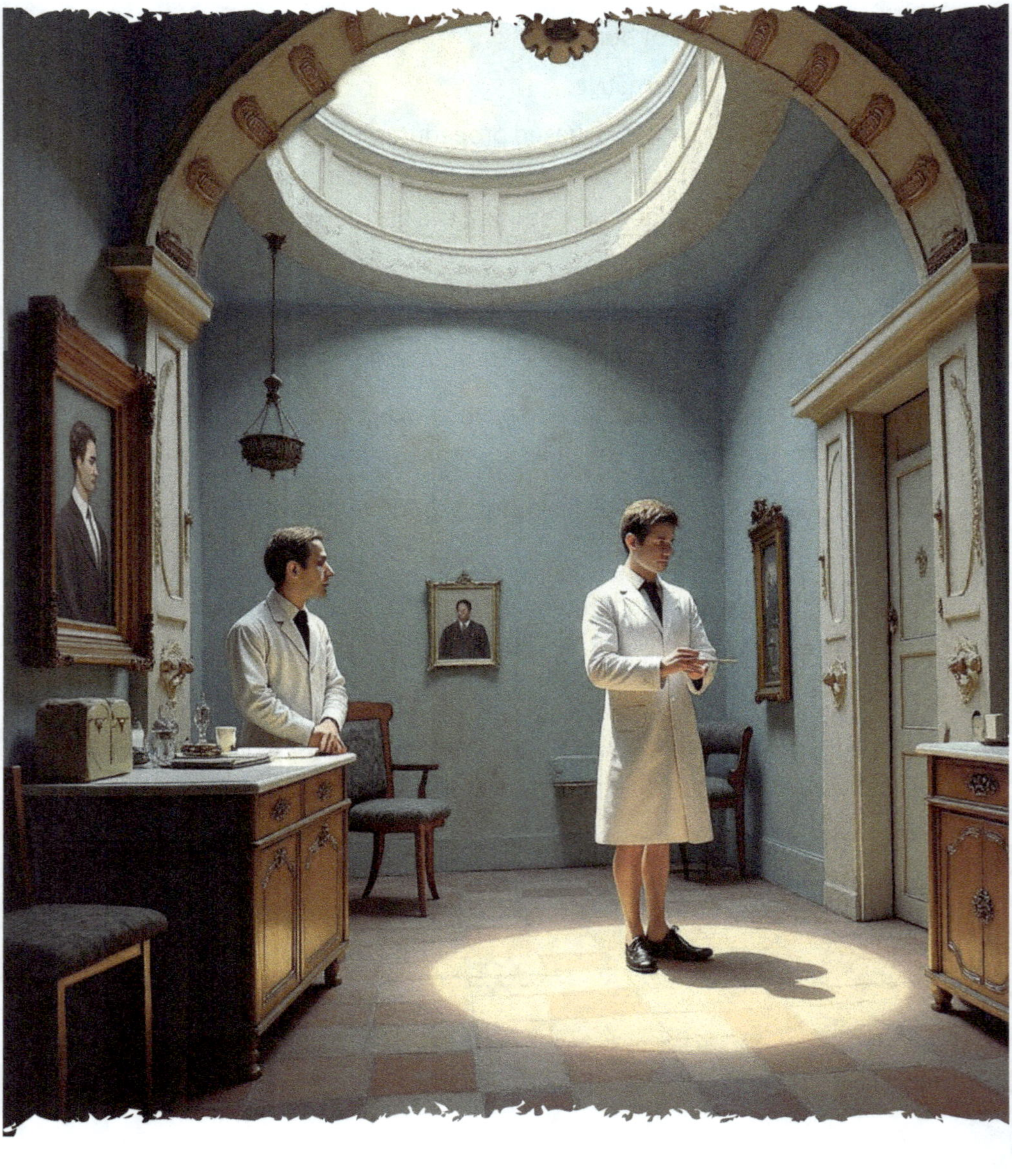

7

CHAPTER

Shaker 1

A Shakespearean Scene in Ten Healing Minutes (Just like an ART treatment):

1st ACT:

Title: The Redeeming of the Tooth

Dramatis Personae:

Dentist (*A zealous, drill-happy practitioner, speaks in monotone couplets*)
Client (*A wary soul, desperate for gentle care, speaks in prose*)
Dental Assistant (*A beleaguered intermediary, speaks in blank verse*)

ACT I, SCENE I

(*A dental chair. The Client reclines, white-knuckling the armrests.
The Dentist looms.*)

Dentist:
"Upon this day,
thy molar needs more room!
Lo, yonder cavity -
A gaping tomb!"

Client:
"No, no, good sir -
I beg thee, be not rash!
I'll take a poultice,
or a honeyed mash.

Must every cure be wrought
with steel and flame?
Doest thou know not
the way more tame?"

(*Enter the Dental Assistant, bearing a tray of dental tools.*)

Dental Assistant:
"My lord,
the patient quakes,
with unpleasant passion.
Shall you not forestall
this industrial action?"

Dentist:
"Pish!
Nature's laws decree:
All rot must yield
to the crownéd might of mine
own gleaming shield!"

(*He picks up a drill as the Client shrieks.*)

ACT I, SCENE II

(*The Client attempts to flee.*
The Dental Assistant blocks the door.)

Client: (*In prose, frantic*)
"Hark! I am but a humble, fearful man!
My teeth and I have lived in peace since time began!"

Dentist: (*Cutting him off*)
"Peace? Nay, 'twas truce!
A coward's fleeting grace!
Behold thy X-ray -
See the traitor's face?"

(*He thrusts a glowing image aloft.
The Client squints.*)

Client:
"That smudge?
That could be anything!
A shadow! A crumb!"

Dentist:
"'Tis the telling fingerprint!
Thy hour hath come!"

(*The Dental Assistant, moved by pity, intercedes.*)

Dental Assistant:
"Good doctor, stay thy hand!
Recall thy oath:
'First, do no harm' -
Though thou art sorely wroth."

Dentist: (*Pausing a minute*)
"Aright then! A compromise -
a hand curette
Shall treat thy state,
but spare thy coward heart."

(The Client exhales in relief,
as the Dentist tosses the drill into the waste bin. Picks up ART hand-tools instead.)

ACT I, SCENE III

(The treatment concludes. The Client bolts upright)

Client:
"T'was gentle, just as I'd thought.
(To the Dentist)
And is how thou shouldst be taught."

(The Client skips away.)

Dental Assistant:
"Alas, the right way:
Such a smarter path.
We heal the tooth,
and longevity we hath."

(Fade to spring flowers swaying in a verdant field.)

8

CHAPTER

Sovereignty

Core points:

1. Complex tooth structure benefits immensely from a mild approach.
2. Summarizing A.R.T.
3. Preparation of the restoration carries most of the risk.
4. Caries removal gel is both painless and non-toxic.

These several studies that scorch the drill and fill approach are so direct. Why are living teeth being drilled into, as though they're chunks of granite?

Teeth are, in fact, remarkable instruments of biological design that are meant to last a lifetime.

They have a crystalline matrix structure that, besides containing the hardest substance in the body (enamel), is also designed to yield and adapt to biting pressures.

The most ancient dentistry of all respects the teeth completely. It's the hand-tools only approach. It's called ART.

It doesn't harm the teeth because it works with the teeth in a sensitive and intelligent manner. It doesn't use the brute force of mechanical machinery.

We can summarize ART this way:

1. Hand tools only.
2. Caries removal gel.
3. Glass Ionomer restoration composite.

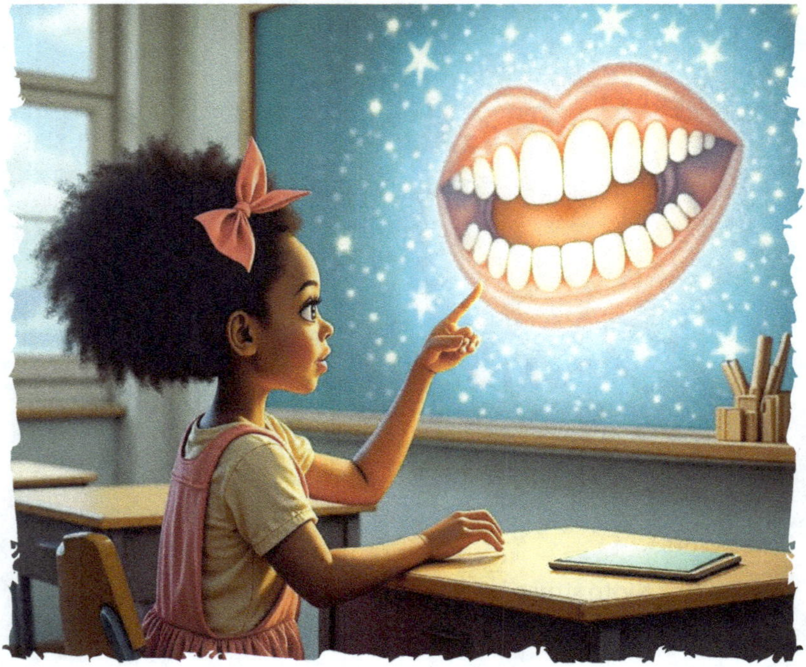

Along with the proper oral hygiene and prevention (good diet included) these three features are in most cases all the reparative method your teeth really need.

The preparation is where most of the damage occurs. Conclusive studies prove that when repair work is done with standard drills, injury happens.

ART prevents this certain injury. It's gentle and stress-free, but it's very effective as well. It's healthier by far. You will actually enjoy your dental visit! You won't be afraid anymore!

Do people really want invasive surgery for their healthy viable teeth? Of course not.

Besides using hand instruments only, ART also employs caries removal gel, which gently and easily dissolves dental decay without any pain, anxiety, or stress.

This is true healing! And your living teeth will live for a very long time!

Medicine should be here to serve. With ART, we get the best of the best. Including a hot drink on the banks of the Elbe, with some of our favorite Rationalists!

9

CHAPTER

Ein Kaffeehaus 1

Title: The Dialectic of Occlusal Margins.

A PLAY IN ONE ACT

Characters:

Dr. Immanuel Kant – A methodical dentist obsessed with moral duty and procedural rigor.

Dr. Arthur Schopenhauer – A brooding, pessimistic dentist who sees pain as inevitable.

Dr. Georg Hegel – An enthusiastic dentist who believes in ART (Atraumatic Restorative Therapy) as the future of dental care.

Setting:

A small Kaffeehaus on the banks of the Elbe. Dresden in the background. Hegel sips a single shot latte, Kant a cappuccino, and Schopenhauer a black espresso.

Hegel: "I must remind you both of liberation. ART is the synthesis dentistry has been waiting for!"

Schopenhauer: "Isn't pain the essence of dental work? All is suffering."

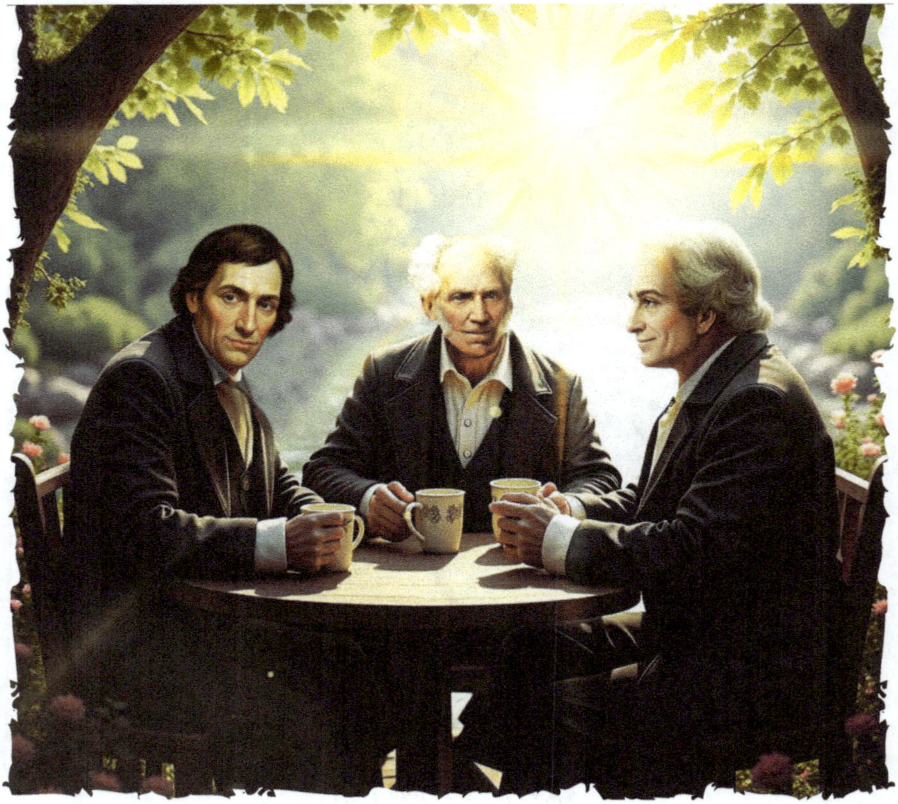

Kant: "Pain is a-posteriori, but our duty is to minimize it through rational principles."

Hegel: "But no more drills. No pain control. Only careful, painless removal of decay, restoring the tooth in harmony with its historical development!"

Schopenhauer: "You coddle the tooth rather than conquer it."

(Hegel places a typodont (a plastic set of teeth) on the table, and proceeds to demonstrate the atraumatic treatment. He knocks over Kant's cup. The drink spills onto Schopenhauer's lap. Kant reaches for the napkin holder and knocks over Hegel's drink.)

Hegel (*ignoring the mess*):

"With the gel, only the decay is removed, leaving the healthy structure intact. A filling is not an imposition but an organic resolution!"

Schopenhauer: "Inevitably there shall be another caries lesion."

Hegel: "Then we advance again! It's the dialectic of dental progress!"

Kant: "The procedure aligns with the categorical imperative of care. As such, it may be morally correct."

Schopenhauer: "The bastards deserve their pain."

Kant: "Nein. I feel truth has triumphed."

Hegel: "Correct. It's the dialectical spur to worldly transcendence."

Schopenhauer: "But you ignore the value of suffering."

Kant: "Duty is the only imperative."

Hegel: "And synthesis. We cannot freeze truth in static dualisms. Today I had to pay two thousand thalers for a light-curing pen."

Kant: "Then you are not grounded in the conditions of possible experience. The light of reason illuminates the categories through which we comprehend phenomena. For example, the non-paying client."

Schopenhauer: "Clients never pay unless we force them. Why else do we overtreat?"

Hegel: "Kant's noumenal realm seems like so much hooey when they don't pay. Still, we must progress dialectically."

Kant: "And maybe you're just being a dummkopf. Ever heard of collection agents?"

Schopenhauer: "Ten million thalers for smile marketing and I still haven't paid off my air compressor."

Hegel: "Kant's thesis/antithesis reveals his struggle with the absolute. Ever tried coercion?"

Schopenhauer: "He doesn't want a lawsuit."

Kant: "Moral law and the dignity of autonomy! You both miss the point!"

Hegel: "Meaning is not found in rigid duty! Only in the dynamic realization of the biomimetic bonding agent."

Schopenhauer: "I tried that once."

Kant: "The categorical imperative that guides rational beings dictates it. You must undertreat and leave remaining viable tissue."

Hegel: "And use Estelite Omega?"

Kant: "In controlled increments!"

Schopenhauer: "You both drown in abstractions. And I'm double parked."

Kant: "Schopenhauer, your pessimism ignores the dignity of autonomy. You still driving that old Audi?"

Hegel: "Gentlemen, doof! Do we have time for historical constructs?"

Kant: "He's right. Look. The waiter wants our money."

10
CHAPTER

Tools

Core points:

1. The A.R.T. toolkit is incredibly economical.
2. A new dental practice using only A.R.T. could be started for a tiny fraction of the usual cost.
3. Dentists would not have huge loans to pay down.
4. Surgical approaches cannot utilize A.R.T. but nearly everything else can.

Atraumatic Restorative Treatment (ART) is most likely the ancient way of doing dentistry. It's by far the most healing way.

ART is nearly 100% painless and does not traumatize the tooth in the many ways that drilling does. It probably suffices for 90% of dental treatments. This is my estimate.

ART requires very modest investment in tools. By manually removing decayed tissue, there are no electric drills, no injections, no damaging thermal and vibrational trauma to living tissues.

Nearly all the trauma of dentistry is alleviated. However, ART tools will not remove existing metal fillings. These will require a special method that I've described in the bonus chapter at the end (Chapter 74.)

Dental colleges sometimes include an ART course in their four-year program. It's presented as an electricity-free option.

Obviously, it's not taken very seriously as a primary approach to dentistry. It needs to be the PRIMARY APPROACH. The real dentistry.

Let's take a look at the very economical ART toolkit:

1. A DiagnoDent, or similar laser-based caries detection method. I'm putting this first because it diagnoses with a much higher accuracy than a traditional manual "prod and poke" method, with a metal explorer.
2. Mouth mirror. Ideally it will have a strong pen light attached. Allows for accurate identification and treatment, especially in the back molar areas. It also serves to retract cheek and tongue for very accurate work.
3. Combination of: Explorer / CPI probe. The CPI probes (cleansing periodontal indicator) scrape away biofilms and plaque. However, probing into deeper gum pockets can carry significant risk of unintended injury via bacterial introduction or damage to sensitive surfaces. Much care is needed.
4. Caries removal gel. This is mostly ignored by conventional dentistry and I will focus on it in-depth at Chapter 40. It's an ultra-beneficial game-changer. CR gel does all the prep-work with zero risk!
5. Isolation Materials. Cotton rolls and rubber dam (if needed).
6. Spoon excavators (small & large). A do-all hand tool for the serious dental healer!
7. Hatchet or dental hoe (for wider cavities and shaping of hard enamel).
8. Dental tweezers. For safety transferring materials.
9. Wedges and strips (for proximal restorations).
10. Glass ionomer cement (GIC). This filling bonds chemically, is biocompatible, and durable. Fuji IX is a popular brand.
11. Mixing pad and spatula. To properly mix the GIC powder and water into an ideal paste.
12. Plastic applier. For accurate GIC placement.
13. Petroleum jelly. For protecting the restoration after placement.
14. Finishing strips (for interproximal surfaces), hand polishing files (optional, for smoothness).

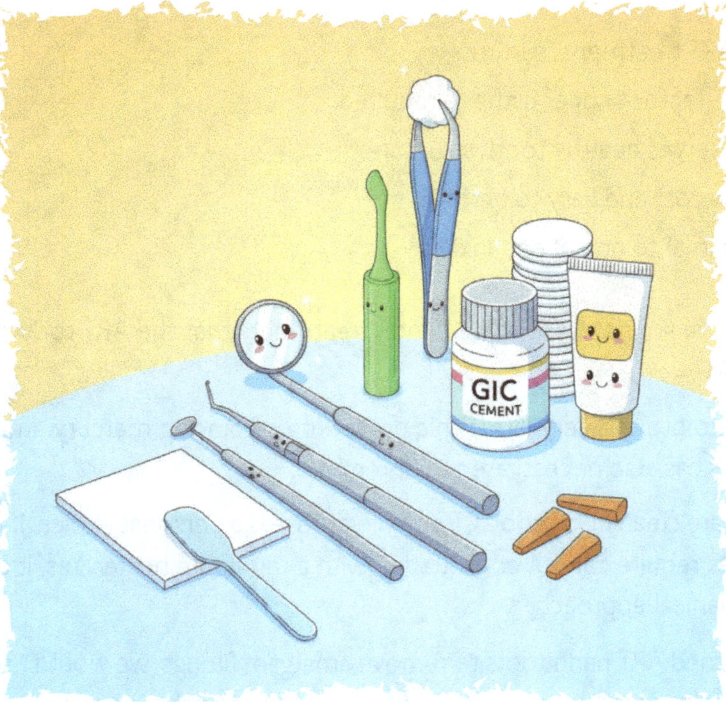

This is your very economical toolkit for excellent restorations.

The typical 50,000 to 200,000 dollar investment for equipping a basic modern dental operatory has now been turned into a well-under 1,000 dollars of basic required equipment for the ART dental healing spa!

Just add a very comfortable client chair that only needs to recline slightly, to ensure maximum comfort and enjoyment, for this pain-free, stress-free treatment!

The results that this ART treatment delivers are also many times healthier!

This ART toolkit would suffice for most basic dental restoration needs. More complex procedures are also feasible using the ART protocol, but I will go into better detail shortly.

The ART treatment features:

1. No electricity or anesthesia required.
2. Preserves healthy tooth structure.
3. Low cost and easy to perform.
4. Minimal to no patient anxiety.

Now the sobriety. Are there dental treatments that the ART toolkit cannot do?

Regrettably, the very iatrogenic procedure of placing mercury amalgam fillings has also necessitated their removal.

They are clearly poisonous. Removing these is a personal choice. If done, it does require careful consultation with a reputable healer. Yes, it uses a mechanical approach.

If we tried ART hand tools to remove amalgam fillings, we would risk further damaging the compromised tooth walls and other dental structure.

Drilling, despite its harm, is still the most viable option in this case. Every precaution is taken to minimize the damage.

Safe amalgam removal is discussed in Chapter 75. It's a controversial area because the Huggins protocol is still not officially approved, even though it tries to make safety its highest priority.

Mechanical drills are actually meant for roads, bridges, trucks. Your living teeth deserve much better!

Mrs. Groves proved it. She expected the worst, and ended up with the best!

11

CHAPTER

O' Neill

Title: An Epiphany

A ONE-ACT PLAY AFTER EUGENE O'NEILL

Characters:
Dr. Horace Whitmore – A middle-aged dentist, weary and disillusioned, haunted by the sound of drills.
Mrs. Eleanor Groves – A nervous patient, late 50s, with a deep fear of dentists.
Lucy – A bright-eyed dental assistant, early 30s, hopeful and progressive.

Setting:
A dimly lit dental office, the walls a sterile white, the air thick with antiseptic and regret. The hum of an old drill lingers like a ghost.

ACT I

(The stage is silent save for the distant whir of a drill in another room. Dr. Whitmore stands at the window, staring at the sun, his hands trembling slightly. Lucy organizes instruments, watching him.)

Lucy: *(softly)*
"You've been quiet today, Doctor."

Whitmore: *(without turning)*
"How many teeth have I drilled in my life, Lucy? Ten thousand? Twenty?"

Lucy:
"I couldn't say."

Whitmore:
"And how many of them needed it?"

(*A pause. The drill in the other room stops abruptly. Silence.*)

Lucy:
"You've helped people."

Whitmore: (*bitter laugh*)
"Have I? Or have I just been... a mechanic of pain?"

(*The door creaks open. Mrs. Groves enters, clutching her purse like a shield.*)

Mrs. Groves:
"I—I'm here for my filling."

Whitmore: (*forcing cheer*)
Ah, Mrs. Groves. Of course.

(*She sits in the chair, gripping the armrests. Whitmore picks up the drill, hesitates. Lucy watches him closely.*)

Lucy: (*quietly*)
"We could try ART."

Whitmore: (*sharply*)
"What?"

Lucy:
"Atraumatic Restorative Treatment. No drilling. Just hand instruments, glass ionomer."

Mrs. Groves: (*hopeful, fearful*)
"No... drill?"

(*Whitmore stares at the drill in his hand, then at Mrs. Groves' terrified face. A long silence.*)

Whitmore: (*whispers*)
"My God."

(*He sets the drill down. It clatters against the tray like a gun being unloaded.*)

ACT II

Whitmore: (*suddenly animated, feverish*)
"Lucy - get the hand excavators. The gel."

Lucy: (*grinning, moving quickly*)
"Yes, Doctor."

Mrs. Groves: (*uncertain*)
"Is this… safe?"

Whitmore: (*fervent, almost manic*)
"Safer than what I've been doing. Safer than cracking teeth open like walnuts."

(*Lucy prepares the caries removal gel. Whitmore leans close to Mrs. Groves, his voice low, urgent.*)

Whitmore:
"Do you know how long we've been drilling? Centuries. Centuries of pain. And for what?"

Mrs. Groves: (*whispers*)
"I don't know."

Whitmore: (*laughs, near-hysterical*)
"Neither do I!"

(*He begins working, carefully applying the gel, removing decay with gentle precision. Mrs. Groves slowly relaxes.*)

Mrs. Groves:
"It… doesn't hurt."

Whitmore: (*voice breaking*)
"No. It doesn't."

ACT III

(The procedure is finished. Mrs. Groves sits up, touching her tooth in wonder.)

Mrs. Groves:
"That's it?"

Whitmore: (softly)
"That's it."

(She looks at him, tears in her eyes.)

Mrs. Groves:
"I've been afraid my whole life."

(Whitmore turns away, overcome. Sobs quietly. Lucy places a hand on his shoulder.)

Lucy:
"You just changed everything."

(Whitmore, regaining composure, stares at the drill on the counter - once his most trusted tool, now a relic of barbarism.)

Whitmore: (to himself)
"The drill is finished."

(The lights fade as the sound of birds outside replaces the memory of the drill's whine. A new day dawns.)

(Curtain)

12

CHAPTER

Longevity

Core points:

1. Who designs the dental college curriculum?
2. Why A.R.T. works best.
3. The benefits of good oral health.
4. The benefits of discussing dental longevity.

ART is the artistic approach to dental longevity. Exactly what people need. I met dozens of dentists and insisted on it. Finally I found a dentist willing to try it. Things have never been the same since.

ART treatment is exactly how to lengthen the lifespan of the teeth to the best extent possible.

I've personally had multiple experiences of dentists diagnosing a "terminal treatment" (a root canal) for what was really a simple ART restoration. Invasive technology is sown into the fabric of the profession.

The writers of the standard dental college curriculum are the national accrediting "bodies":

1. U.S.: Commission on Dental Accreditation (CODA, under the ADA).
2. UK: General Dental Council (GDC).
3. Europe: European Federation of Periodontology (EFP) and national boards.

Along with the dental schools and their senior faculty, and key "influencers", for example:

1. American Dental Association (ADA) – Pushes evidence-based standards.
2. Corporate Interests (eg., Dentsply, Align Tech) – Fund research/equipment that shapes curricula (e.g., CAD/CAM, Invisalign).
3. Academic leaders - Reformulate curricula.

Going deep into this web, you end up with the business structure. That's all we really need to know. It's quite similar to regular medicine, and why shouldn't it be?

If you're going to take serious shots at this structure, then you might end up like Asclepios. Zeus basically threw a thunderbolt at Asclepios. It was a hard judgment.

The result was that all his fabulous healing temples became strip malls.

We need to be careful. Zeus is a tough load. And thunderbolts are no fun, especially coming right after a hot latte and a great conversation on minimally invasive techniques.

ART is radically minimalist but it's also the ancient proven way. When I approached many dozens of dentists to request ART treatment. Even the holistic dentists were reluctant to set aside the drill.

When I finally found a dentist willing to try the ART approach, I supplied the caries removal gel. I carry the stuff just to show the dentists I meet. Nearly all of them have never heard of it!

Caries removal gel is completely pain-free and highly effective. I guess that's why the dentists don't use it!

It works, it's pain-free, and it has no side effects. Skip ahead to Chapter 40 if you want to find out more.

Currently I would estimate that 99.9% of dentists will only use the high-speed drill for caries treatment. Give or take a micron. Those are not very good odds for not being injured by your treatment! Terrible odds in fact.

Having nice healthy teeth is certain to make you much happier. Here are some of the ways:

1. You smile more.
2. You spend less.
3. The rest of your body is better (focal theory)
4. You feel more confident.
5. You worry less.
6. You basically become much more successful!

Success is a subject that's widely written about. Who could ever guess that by ditching painful, scary, injurious dentistry, and replacing it with safe, relaxing, and healthy dentistry, you could be much more successful. But, it's true!

How are you going to get those nice healthy teeth? Certainly with good oral hygiene. But when you must visit a dentist, will you get healing or injury? It's a key question we need to ask.

Having a lucid conversation on tooth longevity with a dentist is one path to clarity. Expect to make frequent corrections. The four-year program he took doesn't promote it.

The dentist was mostly trained in repairs. That's why it's a challenge. Longevity is a different animal.

Hopefully, we're rewriting an entire paradigm. Even rewriting history, if a legendary playwright has anything to say about it!

13

CHAPTER

A Trade Fair

Core points:

1. A large dental trade show offers unique opportunities to ask strategic questions about dental healing.

I recently attended a dental trade fair, a two-day event at a large convention center.

The admission was 500 dollars. That's serious money if you're a healer. Not so much if you're making a fortune selling new technologies to the industry.

Dentistry is very lucrative. Several of the booths offered coaching on practice profit optimization.

I devised a scale, from 0 to 100, with 0 being for ideal health and wellness, and 100 for absolute profitability. I asked the vendors to rate themselves on this scale.

Several times, I thought I was going to be attacked with expensive dental appliances. Or doused with patented oral rinses.

However, some of the vendors readily grasped the idea of dental longevity. They loved this focus.

One booth in particular was paying cash to dentists for their gold-filled extractions. These dental entrepreneurs really understood alluvial placer mining.

I wondered if the patients were ever consulted on this lucrative trade. This was not a welcome line of inquiry.

The open bar started at 5 pm. It was very crowded. Drinks flowed and everyone seemed happy about the industry.

I started asking if any booths were offering the very healthy and painless caries removal gel made from papaya enzyme.

This question made people nervous. I was going against the pain and trauma culture.

So I one-upped with questions about how endodontic (root canal) bacterial risks could be mitigated, ideally with Ozone treatment.

I even had the audacity to suggest that in a large majority of these cases, the tooth could be saved.

People were not laughing anymore, so I had to come up with dental jokes, fast.

I pretended I was a German rationalist philosopher who had recently obtained a dental degree.

Now they started laughing again. They even liked my fake accent.

People ordered more beer and wine. They wanted to know more about the radical concepts I was offering! Where did I find out about this kind of healing?

So I mentioned the Tooth Fairy. She is a staunch supporter of Atraumatic Dentistry.

Maybe she wrote the book on it. Currently, she's somewhere in China, searching for the missing Wei Jing (see Chapter 43).

When she finds it, dentistry will be even better. A new curriculum will emerge, one that puts the client's interest ahead of the profession's. That day can't come too soon.

Dental conventions are a lot of fun. Provided you have 500$ to spare. Otherwise, you have to infiltrate it for free by being a bartender, or... a Tooth Fairy!

14

CHAPTER

The ART Roadmap

Core points:

1. Step by step on how to provide an A.R.T. treatment.
2. A.R.T. could be learned by many types of care providers.
3. The less done invasively to teeth, the healthier they will be.

Question: What is rarer than a 10 ounce bar of pure gold lying on a busy street?

Answer: A dentist willing to set aside his power-turbines and do a much healthier and virtually painless ART restoration!

But not for long! We are here to change the entire game! And change it, we will!

Here is a step by step tutorial on how to do an excellent atraumatic restoration:

1. Chat with your client to make sure they understand that there will be NO stress and NO pain!
2. Seat them comfortably.
3. Isolate the Tooth: Clean and dry the tooth and place cotton wool rolls to absorb saliva.

4. Using the smallest suitable excavator, widen the cavity entrance just enough to allow instrument access.
5. Apply the caries removal gel. Let it dissolve the caries in minutes. Repeat until it stops turning cloudy.
6. Gently remove soft, infected dentin.
7. With the sharp spoon-shaped excavator, carefully scrape away the soft, wet, and demineralized dentin. The technique relies on feeling the difference in hardness.
8. Leave the hardest discolored "affected" dentin. This layer is demineralized but not infected and can remineralize, so it is left in place.
9. Clean the prepared cavity with a wet cotton pellet, then a dry one to remove any debris.
10. Optional: Condition the enamel and dentin surfaces for a few seconds using a dentin conditioner (usually a weak polyacrylic acid) provided with the GIC. This cleans the surface and improves the bond.
11. Rinse the conditioner off thoroughly with a wet cotton pellet, ensuring no residue remains.
12. Dry the cavity gently with dry cotton pellets. The cavity should be moist but not wet; a glistening surface is ideal.
13. Hand-mix the Glass Ionomer Cement (GIC) powder and liquid to a smooth, creamy consistency within the recommended working time (usually 30-45 seconds).
14. Insert the mixed GIC into the cavity in small increments using an appenser/carrier instrument. Press and condense the material firmly into the cavity and against the walls using a slightly overfilled, petroleum-jelly-coated gloved finger. This is called the "finger-press" technique and ensures a good seal.
15. After the material has set slightly (usually 1-2 minutes), ask the patient to bite down on articulating paper to check the bite. Remove any high spots with a carver.
16. Finally, apply a protective layer of petroleum jelly over the restoration and advise the patient not to eat for at least one hour.

This basic protocol should only be done by a trained ART practitioner.

However, you get the idea: it's elegant, simple, highly effective, stress-free.

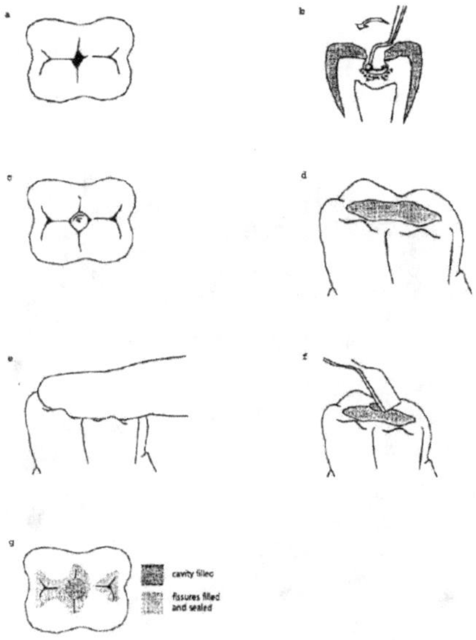

Key points:

1. Minimal Intervention: Remove only what is necessary.
2. Hand Instruments Only: No electricity or drills needed.
3. Adhesive Material: Uses a material that bonds to the tooth and releases fluoride.
4. Patient Comfort: A virtually painless procedure, usually eliminating the need for anesthesia.

Truly, the less you do to the vital living teeth, the healthier they will be!

Does modern dentistry like it when you keep coming back for more repairs? And do you keep coming because of what modern dentistry does?

A very scary concept!

ART is a core skill that could be learned by many types of health professionals.

It could be learned in only a few days. I will soon describe how I was tutored in doing a basic composite restoration. I learned it in two hours.

ART promises healthy treatments with no trauma. Only very few treatments, usually involving surgery, are beyond its range. It's THE game changer!

Now we need to book a long ocean cruise quickly! We have some very LOUD singing to do!

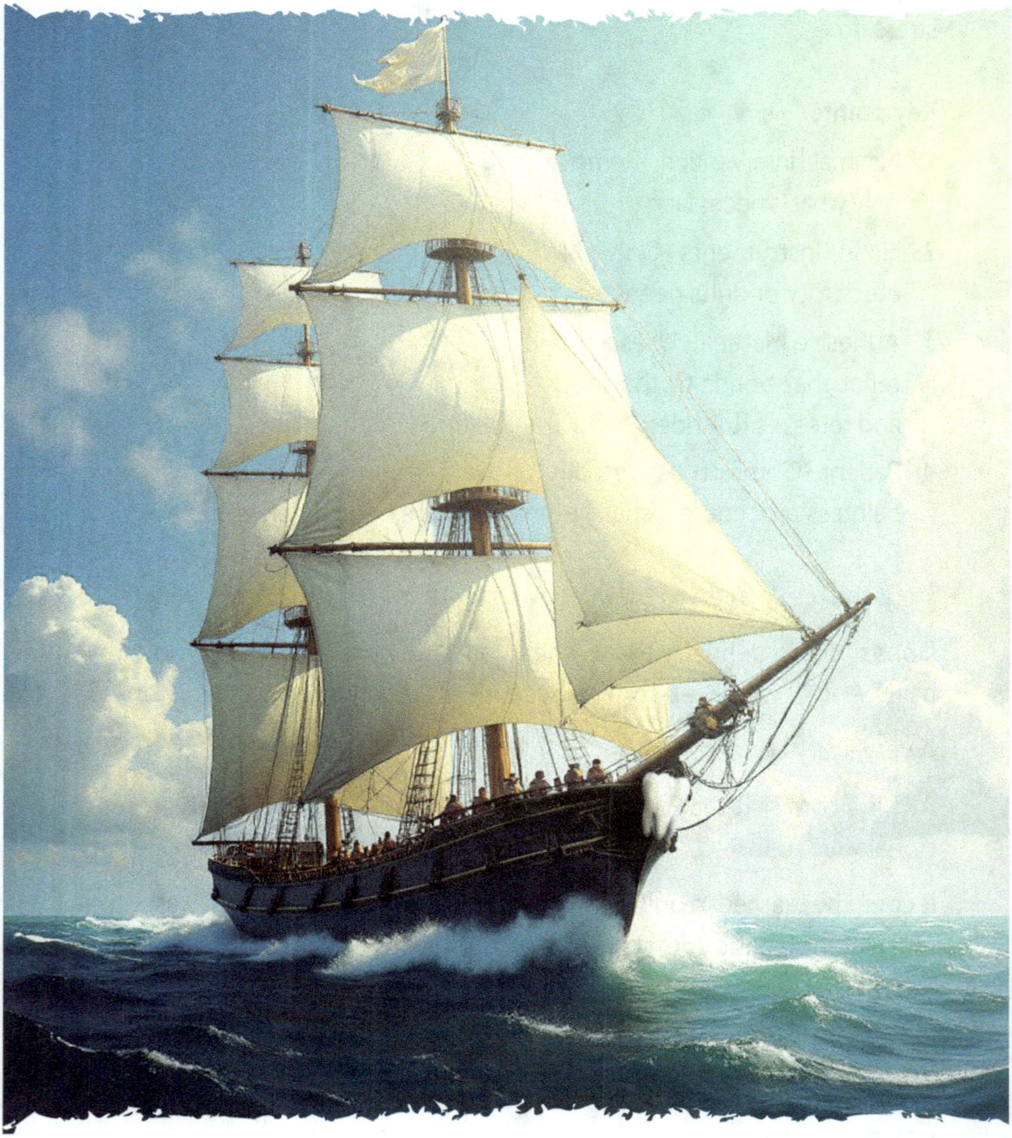

15

CHAPTER

Bosun DDS

In the ancient times, the mariners worked real hard, swabbing decks, mending nets, scraping barnacles, and other… um… stuff.

They needed good music and the sea shanty turned toil into some good time fun!

It bred camaraderie as workers would outdo each other for loudness. Shanty comes from the French "chanter", to sing. It's actually shouting, though:

Title: The Ballad of Bosun DDS

(VERSE I)

Oh gather ye round, ye scoundrel mess,
And hear of Bosun DDS,
Minimally invasive that heals yer state,
And leaves ya calm and peaceful, mate!

(CHORUS)

Then ho! Ho! For the clever hand,
That saves the tooth and spares the man!
We'll sing for ART both night and day,
And keep the drill locked far away!

(VERSE 2)

The new ways spray like gentle rain,
That cure the wrong and ease the pain,
Now we fix the caries so swift,
It's gonna give yer a mighty lift!

(CHORUS)

Then ho! Ho! For the glass so bright,
That seals the tooth up good and tight!
No cannon's roar nor shot nor shell,
Just clean, quick work - and done so well!

(VERSE 3)

Ye captains proud with golden teeth,
Ye cabin boys with limited means,
Come seek the doc who heals with ease,
And saves yer smiles upon the seas!

(FINAL CHORUS - LOUD!)

Then ho! HO! Let the chorus ring,
For dentists, smart and that's the thing!
Them drills may sleep in Davy's hold,
As we keep yer teeth from growing old!

(TOOT TOOT! SPIT-SPIT!)

[This ribald tune has been endorsed by the Committee for Responsible Shanty Swigging.]

16

CHAPTER

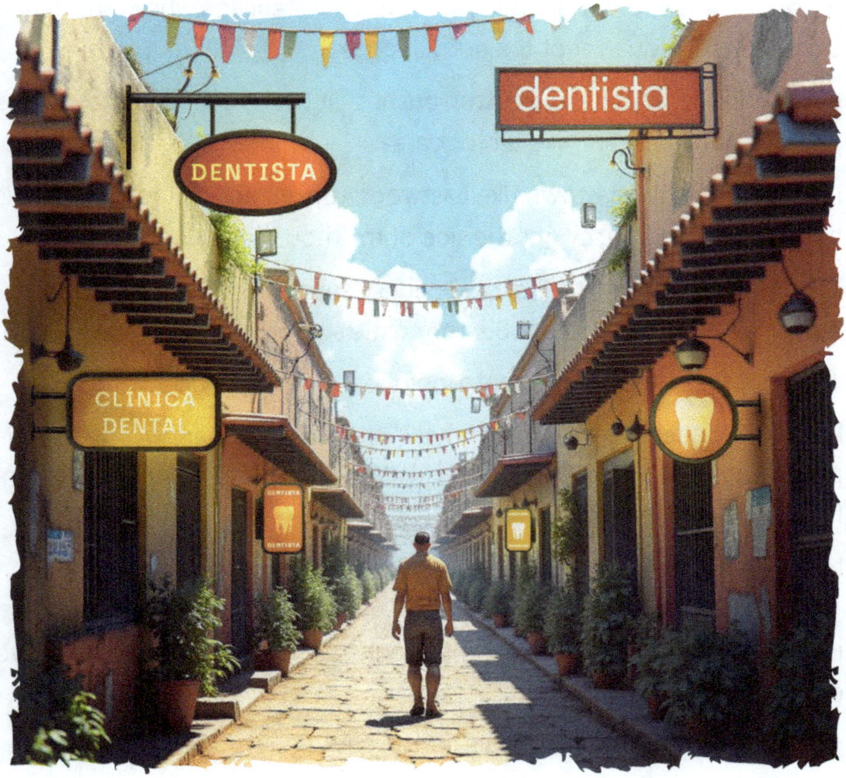

The Search

Core points:

1. The challenge of finding a hands-only willing dentist.
2. Why invasive dentistry is so entrenched.
3. Guiding an endodontist through an A.R.T.-only treatment.

The ART of dental healing replaces the sense of dread and anxiety with peacefulness and confidence.

Not so long ago I found myself in a Mexican border town called Los Algodones. This town is a nexus for North Americans who want dental treatments at a quarter of the normal price.

Los Algodones means "the cotton bushes". It has over 300 dental offices packed tightly in a ten square block area.

I arrived in that dusty town like Eastwood looking for a place to park his burro. I spit some baccy out the side of my mouth.

Then I began talking with the local trade. Cautiously at first. I insisted that I be treated ONLY with hand tools, the gentle age-old method known as ART.

The dentists all replied "lo siento, no puedo".... "sorry, no can do..."

I deeply wondered why none of these professionals were willing to simply unplug their drilling turbine and just do a basic hands-only restoration. It should be so straightforward!

I retreated often to the local bistro to ponder why.

Here are some of the reasons that dentists are "stuck" on very invasive dentistry and remain there:

1. They're heavily trained in pain and anxiety.
2. It's the result of four years of dental college training.
3. It's a science-first curriculum.
4. It doesn't actually teach healing (not part of the course content).
5. The dentist goes deeply into debt (unless coming from a wealthy family or being a lottery winner).
6. The focus is all on power tools and scientific biology.
7. When the dentist graduates he needs to pay that debt down fast.
8. The start up equipment and new premises costs are very high.
9. They're expected to be "professional" and have a very nice lifestyle. (entry barriers are high)

10. The quick turnaround of clients ensures an easy daily shift.
11. Insurance rewards them for invasive treatments.
12. And mostly: the customers never question any of it!
13. Even though it's quite likely injurious.

ART is an entirely different kind of dentistry. Undentistry!

After a disappointing week, I arrived at the door of a curandero disguised as an invasive endo.

When that one dentist finally agreed to treat me with hand tools only, I think he hadn't had a customer all week.

He was an older fellow with the middle name "del Dios". (Of God). Small cues are like bread crumbs and you follow them assiduously.

First, we used the caries removal gel that I'd brought with me. I travel with two packs of it. Sorry. I'm just a travelling obsessed dental healer. It's the hat I wear.

He didn't have any CR gel but he was amazingly interested in it. He applied it and it worked like magic. The way it's supposed to.

The "papatine-based" gel causes decay to mush up and become soft. After a minute, it removes easily. 100% painless, as you might imagine.

He applied it three or four times. Until all the soft decay was gone. He finished by using the hand tool called the curette (there are around 6 of these hand tools in ART) to scrape the remaining decay.

He pushed a bit hard, so I gently reminded him, "Easy, easy. Don't push with force, just peck like a chipmunk or a woodpecker". He got it.

Finally, the restoration was clean and ready. He used the light-cured composite method, which is not the traditional ART way. ART usually uses glass-ionomer cement (GIC). However, he didn't have any GIC on hand.

He applied the etching liquid first (an acid), which results in a porous surface for the composite to stick to.

He washed and dried it off. Then he applied a coat of (super-glue type) dental adhesive with a tiny brush that looks like a makeup brush.

Then he applied the composite in thin layers. The composite has to be light cured for each thin layer. It's 20 seconds of a bright blue laser-light. That's why there's an orange plastic cover over the pen. To neutralize the blue light.

The layer has to be below a certain thickness, otherwise it won't cure and set properly. It would be soft in the middle, which means a ruined restoration.

Applying the composite is very "technique sensitive". Good technique equals a good restoration that lasts a very long time.

At the end of the treatment, he reached for his power tool to do the polishing. NO senor. This is 100% hand tools. Sin comprometer.

So we did the polishing by hand as well.

IT WAS PERFECT.

The entire treatment was a revelation. No pain, no stress, just ease and comfort.

And did I actually hear this old fellow whistling while he was working? That would probably be the first time in his career.

Have you ever heard a dentist whistle while he works?

You will in the future, after you toss harmful mainstream dentistry and switch to ART!

This little episode in a tiny village of Mexican dentists proved beyond any doubt that safe, effective, painless, and healthy dental treatment is far superior to the drill-based invasive kind.

It's painless, stress-free, relaxing, and even enjoyable.

AND… it's much healthier! MUCH healthier. Time to PARTY!

Now, it's just a matter of time until the reservoir of truth percolates back up to the surface, the way it was for many hundreds of years.

It's been there in ancient libraries the whole time. But those libraries were dimensional. They were not normal libraries, that's for certain…

17

CHAPTER

Cruz del Sur

A REFLECTION AFTER J.L. BORGES

A librarian in Buenos Aires heard it from a man who once treated a patient who claimed to have been present at the invention of the drill.

"In the unfathomable archives of human suffering, there exists a dark and branching corridor. A via dolorosa of enamel and nerve.

"For centuries, men with steel instruments (descendants, perhaps, of very angry doctors) believed that to cleanse a tooth, one must first wound it.

"The anesthetic needle and high-speed turbine were their chosen implements, a method that turned the mouth into a battleground.

"I have seen patients enter those chambers white-knuckled, gripping the arms of the chair as if it were the edge of a precipice. They emerged shaken, their teeth saved, yes, but their memory of the ordeal etched deeper than any filling.

"Then, like a whisper in the infinite Library of Babel, another way appeared. It came not from the grand halls of European dentistry, but from the quiet pragmatism of those who worked in places where electricity was a luxury, and pain a needless extravagance.

"Atraumatic Restorative Treatment (ART) required no drill, no needle, no conquest. Only a hand steady enough to lift decay as one lifts a page from an ancient manuscript - careful, precise, leaving the structure beneath intact.

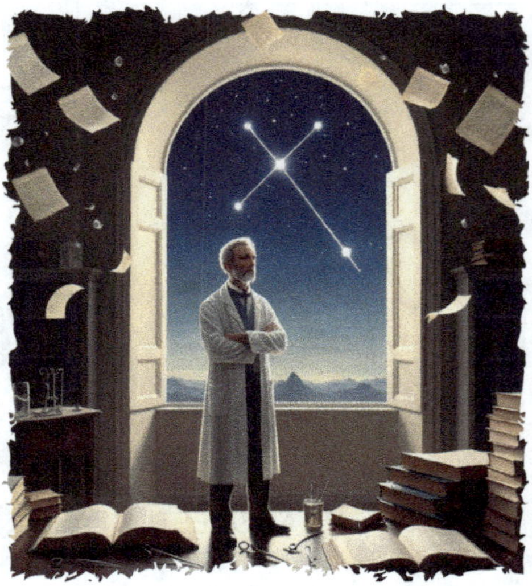

"I once met a dentist in Adrogué who told me this: A tooth is not an enemy. It is a text. Written in calcium and collagen, its history visible in every stain, every fracture. To read it properly, one must not burn the pages.

"He demonstrated ART with the patience of a scribe restoring a palimpsest. The glass ionomer he used was a kind of mirror. Not the cold, reflective kind, but the sort that absorbs and becomes part of what it touches.

"Now, the old ways persist in places, like echoes of a dream no one remembers dreaming. But in certain clinics, in certain hands, the violence has been unmasked as superstition.

"A child sits in the chair. There is no scream of machinery. Only the quiet scrape-scrape of a hand instrument, the patient press of cement. The child leaves curious, unharmed. The tooth remains, not conquered, but mended.

"And so the story folds inward, as all good stories do. The drill, once standard of care, now seems destined for the hall of memories best forgotten. ART is not new - it is a rediscovery, a return to the oldest truth: Healing need not be a war.

"I cannot say if ART is the future. But I know it is already the past - a path we forgot, then found again, like a verse misplaced in the universe's endless library."

18
CHAPTER

E Study

Core points:

1. Dental hygienists are an excellent on-ramp to A.R.T.
2. Drilling shows several injury outcomes.
3. The challenge of saying No to drills.

Good news: It turns out that ART is being selectively taught to dental hygienists in certain jurisdictions. I wonder if some elements don't like the idea of ART going fully mainstream. HA. We shall see about that!

ART means that you never have to be subjected to regular terrifying dentistry again. Imagine that.

For one, your treatments might all be done by the hygienist, saving you a fortune. This is assuming you don't have any terminal-dental issues. In which case, yes, do go to a regular dentist because they all do surgery anyway.

But for basic restorations and things like cleaning and prevention advice, a hygienist could fill all your needs.

Let's look at another key study. In 2003, Professor Richard Elderton investigated the long-term harms of excessive dental drilling (which reinforced Brännström's earlier study).

Key findings:

1. Each drill-and-fill cycle weakens teeth, leading to larger restorations, then crowns, then extractions.

2. 60–70% of fillings replaced were clinically avoidable if minimally invasive approaches were used.
3. Dentists often drill beyond decayed areas ("extension for prevention"), sacrificing healthy tooth structure.
4. Over-drilled margins increase gaps, letting bacteria cause recurrent decay.
5. Aggressive drilling creates micro-fractures that grow under chewing forces.
6. Even "shallow" drills risk pulpitis due to heat/vibration (echoing Brännström 1965).
7. Over-cut dentin compromises bond strength of modern adhesives.
8. Drilled teeth are more brittle, prone to cracks under normal biting. (The tooth's sensitive crystalline matrix is seriously harmed).
9. Replacing failed fillings costs 3–5x more than early, conservative care. (ie: ART).
10. At dental school students learn mechanical prep skills but not biological preservation.
11. Excessive drilling leads to lifetime of repairs, reducing tooth longevity.
12. ART (Atraumatic Restorative Treatment) and air abrasion outperform drills in all cases.
13. Drilling is often a short-term (easy) fix with long-term costs.

These studies are....well, disruptive is not even the word for it. How about... annihilating? Hmmm... even that's too mild.

Why do dentists use drills?

1. Speed
2. Insurance incentives
3. Outdated dental education

With ART we turn the "lose-lose" into the "win-win". So easy. It all starts with saying NO, very empathically. NO to wrong treatment.

After a while, saying NO to terrifying dentistry will be the most fun we'll ever have.

Mechanical drills whirr at 300,000 rpm, and teeth experience significant trauma. The large hypodermic needles are no laughing matter either. They are also not needed with ART.

UNDENTISTRY... Deconstructing in order to rebuild.

"Built on a foundation

Of happy truth, not terror.

Solutions often happen

When we say no to error."

There's debate about whether those Wild West days were genuine, or were they mostly created in movie studios?

Regardless, the lone western hero does show up unexpectedly as a healer of teeth! The sheriff didn't expect that!

19

CHAPTER

Grit

Setting: A scorched desert town, where the only thing drier than the riverbeds are the townsfolk's gums.

The wind howls through the empty streets, carrying the distant whirrrr of outlaw drills. A lone figure rides into town- Dr. Clint Eastooth as "The dentist with no name," his ART kit strapped to his saddle like a gunslinger's arsenal.

Inside, a group of roughnecks wince as black-hatted dentist Lee VanTeeth leans over a screaming patient, his steam-powered drill roaring like a locomotive. Clint steps in, his shadow stretching long across the floor.

VanTeeth: (*looking over*) "This town's got only one kind of dentist, stranger." (*revs drill menacingly*)

Dr. Eastooth: (*spits tobacco*) "Yeah. The wrong kind."

(*The saloon falls silent. The patient whimpers. Clint's hand hovers near his air abrasion wand.*)

VanTeeth: "Heard the rumors about you. You really think your fancy painless tricks can beat real dentistry?"

Dr. Eastooth: "A man's mouth oughta be his own… not your damn battleground."

(*VanTeeth grimaces as the client bolts for the door*)

Dr. Eastooth: "You're scaring folks, VanTeeth."

VanTeeth: (*grins, revving drill*) "Pain's how they learn."

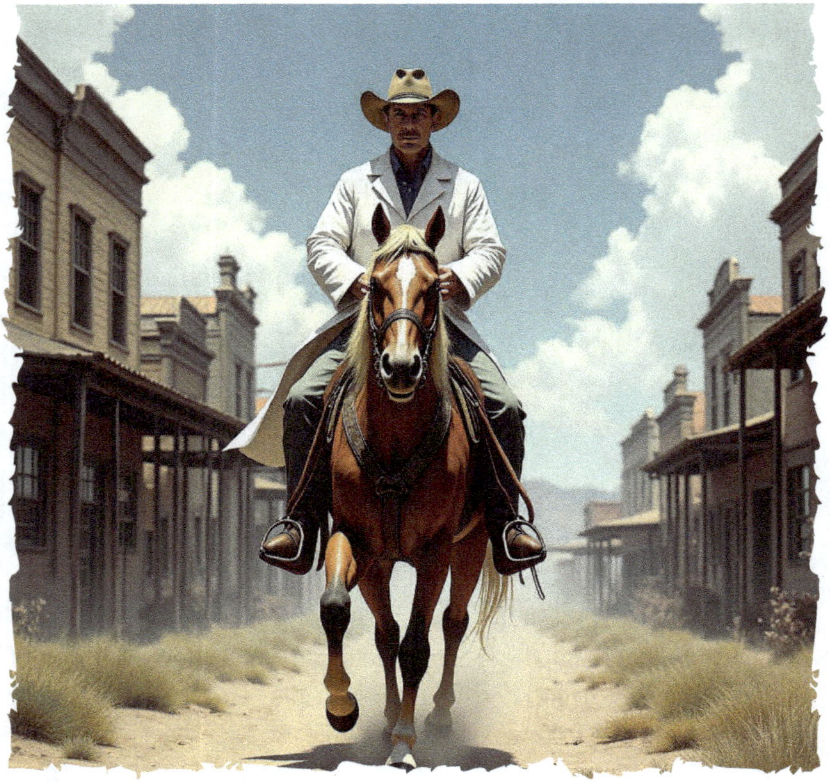

Dr. Eastooth snatches up his light curing pen and VanTeeth freezes.

Dr. Eastooth: (*snarls*) "Go ahead. Make my filling."

(*long pause*)

Dr. Eastooth: "Respect ain't born from fear. Now fix their damn teeth right."

VanTeeth: (*grimacing*) "Stranger, you got yourself a lot of swag."

Dr. Eastooth: (*glaring intensely*) "I earned that swag. Now you just gonna watch me save all these folks' teeth, or are you gonna help?"

VanTeeth: (*glares, but slightly less intensely*) "I don't make new deals easy. But looks like you got something going here."

Dr. Eastooth: (*spits tobacco*) "You're damn right I do!"

Eastooth became legend.
His legacy lives on in ART.

20

CHAPTER

Risk *Management*

Core points:

1. Managing the risks in dental treatment is very smart.
2. A hobbit analogy for minimally invasive techniques.
3. Reasons that people avoid dentists.
4. How they try to cope without dental care.

There is obviously a lot of risk in dentistry. Treatments are very seldom mild, and the results are irreversible. You just can't go back and regain lost enamel. Or a tooth lost.

You take your chances. Hopefully, with wisdom, you minimize these risks to near-zero. It's rare but possible.

The rigidity in dentistry can be pulverized, and replaced by common sense and the "will to wellness". Like Hegel and Kant said, it's the dialectic to progress.

Every treatment can be divided into two parts:

1. The preparation
2. The restoration.

The restoration part is mostly straightforward. The dentist fills a clean, well-prepared and treated cavity.

BUT. Nearly all the risk is contained in the preparation part! That's where the dangerous high-speed drills are. It's where needle injections are.

If you could transform that part of dentistry, you probably have a mostly safe treatment. That's the challenge! It's solvable.

The hobbits were very self-reliant folks. Stout and sturdy. Their villages often had just one part-time nurse. They knew how to take care of themselves.

According to legend, this is what they had:

1. Basic ART hand tools.
2. Some caries removal gel (a miracle substance that I will describe soon)
3. Good lighting and a good mirror.
4. Courage which is sourced from common sense.

They would actually do their own prep and leave the restoration (lower risk) part to the dentist! Brilliant!

This way they avoided all needles and drills. Imagine that! So clever.

In the case of deep caries or other problems, then yes, they would seek the best healers.

Most of their food came out of their gardens, so they had few issues to begin with.

When the dentist viewed their excellent preparation (sealed with a temporary filling) he'd be delighted! Those hobbits were so practical.

People avoid dentists because they feel that many things are "wrong" about it. Why should healthcare include terror?

These are actually logical people. Here are the top reasons that people avoid dentists:

1. Fear & Anxiety (Dental Phobia). Amazingly, nearly everyone abhors needles and 300,000 rpm drills into their bodies! Someday the dental colleges (and their curriculum writers) will learn this.
2. Dislike of surgery. Amazingly, dentists work in operatories. This is a place where surgery happens! Someday the curriculum writers will notice this. Wait! They like it that way. Surgery every time. Big power.
3. The sounds and smells of a dental office can trigger anxiety. No kidding. How about the smell of living viable dental tissue being removed for no competent reason. Always terrifying.
4. Dental care can be expensive, especially for procedures like fillings, crowns, or root canals. And paying for something you probably don't need, which is also very harmful and irreversible, is also a "major, mega bummer trip".
5. They lack dental insurance.
6. Some feel that if they don't feel pain, there's no need for a check-up.
7. Bad past experiences. Like, mercury poisoning leading to job loss and chronic fatigue. No way! That would seriously hurt. Plus, expensive as anything!
8. Negative interactions with dentists (feeling judged or rushed). For example "I know because of my four hard years of science, passing my exams, etc. and you don't".
9. Cultural Beliefs (some cultures avoid dentists unless absolutely necessary). For example: "God is protecting me from undue harm".

In the UK, dentistry is so expensive (not to mention, harmful) that many are completely "out of the system" and doing their own dentistry. Yes, it's gotten that bad over there in crumpet land. We will monitor how that goes.

They're simply not getting what they need from mainstream dentistry. Can you blame them?

I've spoken with people who have neglected their dentistry for many years, and their teeth are in very poor condition. However they are simply too terrified of the entire experience to willingly go back. I feel sorry for them.

One chap I met hadn't been to a dentist in 30 years. I asked: "How do you cope?"

"With magnets," he replied.

"Magnets?"

"Yeah. They kill the pain."

That is the saddest damn thing! It's so unnecessary. That's why this book is in your hands!

These kinds of people should ideally start with an empathic and understanding dental hygienist, and go from there. If they knew the existence of ART, their lives would completely change.

The dental avoiders are a unique segment of the general population. They need to be reached with some common sense. They need to know that awesome solutions exist!

[**Disclaimer:** Please run all these legendary Hobbit self-treatment ideas past a qualified and licensed HEALER first. This way, you'll get a more complete picture of how to proceed. There will be no risks at all.]

Now it's time to check back in with our German philosopher-dentists. They're all trained in appropriate standards of care. So we're on very safe ground. Or are we?

21

CHAPTER

Ein Kaffeehaus 2

"A CASUAL DENTAL SYMPOSIUM BY THE RHINE."

Afternoon light slants through the hanging flowerpots on a terrace overlooking the river.

Three dentist-philosophers sit around a round wooden table, each holding a hot kaffeegläser.

Immanuel Kant wears a dental bib to avoid stains. Arthur Schopenhauer stirs his Einspänner while Georg Hegel enjoys the river's historical necessity.

Kant: "Gentlemen, often in dentistry, we have a synthetic judgement a-posteriori, discovered through sensory experience - specifically, pain."

Schopenhauer: "Ah, pain is another word for our craft!"

Hegel: "Correction, Herr Arthur. Pain, and the caries, is an abstract negation. We need Aufhebung, the antithesis, to arrive at a final synthesis!"

Kant: "And is this synthesis atraumatic?"

Schopenhauer: "Better be! The stress! The discomfort! And why?"

Kant: "Not for rationality, that's certain!"

Schopenhauer: "Ja, and if that method causes further injury?"

Hegel: (*stands abruptly*) "Then we invoke the dialectical progression to healing!"

Kant: (*raises an arm, as though to protect himself*) "In all cases it must involve the categorical imperative of the universal law - an Atraumatic Treatment for all rational beings!"

Schopenhauer: "And I shall take a break from excessive rationality and sip a Pilsner."

Hegel: (*turning, pacing*) "Schoppy, reason is the material embodiment of the Concept, consciously shaping reality! We heal! Our fundamental duty!"

Kant: "Correct, Herr Georg. The a-priori elegance of ART synthesizes co-rrupted dentin into the unified experience of the perfect restoration. No pain! No stress! Wunder! Pass the cinnamon, please!"

Schopenhauer: "A triumph of reason! Like reading Spinoza on a quiet afternoon! The methodical removal of erroneous passion, leaving only clear, rational substance! Nutmeg also?"

Hegel: "Dental boards! Pfui! (*snorts into his drink and sprays the others*)

Kant: (*wiping his jacket*) "Corrupted curricula?"

Hegel: (*points skyward*) "Forgetting the Umgreifende, the ALL!"

Schopenhauer: "Seems like a business school…"

Kant: (*with a foam mustache*)
"We cannot deny the categorical imperative! Caries removal gel carries the duty to restore the tooth! And somehow, they ignore it!" (*flicks his teaspoon; it lands on Schopenhauer's lap*)

Hegel: (*gesturing passionately*) "Of course, Herr Emmanuel. They seem almost… afraid of it!"

Schopenhauer: (*fumbling for the spoon*) "Afraid! A simple plant based curative! What kind of….!!"

Kant: (*interrupting*) "They do not always act on rational principles, Herr Arthur."

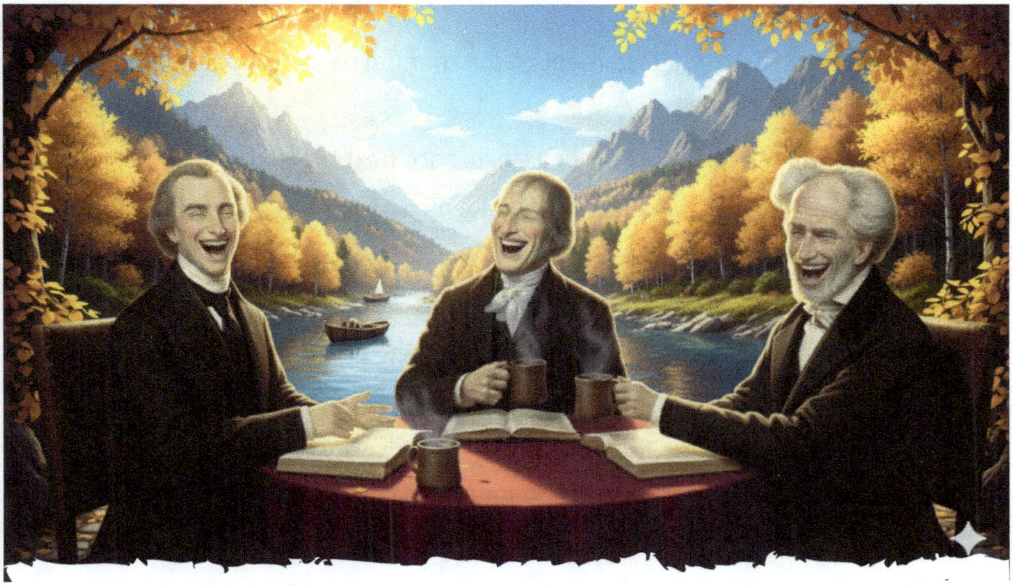

Hegel: (*pacing*) "Also seem afraid of the ozone treatment! Calling it experimental, despite such proven success!"

Kant: "Lacherlich!"

Hegel: (*sitting down very carefully*) "It merely negates the pathological particularity of the microbes, dissolving them into the universal medium of air and water! It is the abstract, universal concept of cleanliness realizing itself in the tooth!" (*slaps the table hard, spilling Kant's drink*)

Schopenhauer: "Merely the cure manifested in biocompatible format. Efficient, rational, and superior! Achieved with profound seriousness! Only seriousness!"

Kant: "You're sure?"

Schopenhauer: "Ja! Excellent not because it is joyful, but because it is NOT terrible!"(*frowns*)

Kant: "Schoppy, even "not terrible" represents an advance for dentistry! Yet, I had expected perhaps a more cheerful adjective..."

Hegel: (*rises abruptly, knocking over Schopenhauer's drink*) "Then I shall supply it! The noumenal synthesis! The tooth now appears as what it truly is: a reconciled unity, a testament to the triumph of the Dental Spirit over material decay!"

Schopenhauer: "He must order a single shot next time!"

Kant: "Gentlemen, we have come to the Poesis! The atraumatic and minimally invasive as Ultimate Geist!"

Hegel: (*pacing, agitated*) "And so, dentistry shall put the client ahead of its own interests! The spirit of dentistry becoming conscious of its true aim at last!"

Schopenhauer: (*rising from the table, knocking over Kant's drink*) "This makes me feel so positive. It's strange! I shall take positive workshops now. Many workshops."

Kant: (*slaps table*) "Even better, Schoppy. You shall participate in the self-realization of the Absolute through the Wunder of Atraumatic Dentistry!"

Hegel: (hopping up and down in joyful abandon) "Nothing less shall do! PROST!"

22

CHAPTER

B1 Study

Core points:

1. Describing drill micro-fracturing
2. How A.R.T. minimizes or negates these risks.
3. The dental college curriculum needs to promote the safest means.
4. Holistic dentistry evolution.

Avijit Banerjee, a London-based dental detective, is one of the important figures in alternative dentistry. The Banerjee study (2000) confirmed nearly all of Brännström's earlier findings:

(**Title:** The effect of rotary instrumentation on dentin microstructure.)

Key Findings:

1. Subsurface microfractures observed in 72% of teeth after high-speed drilling (even with water cooling).
2. Cracks extended 250–400 μm into dentin, often reaching the dentinoenamel junction (DEJ)
3. Microfractures at filling edges increased secondary decay risk by 40%
4. Cracks acted as bacterial highways, correlating with higher RCT (root canal) rates.
5. Conclusion: Rotary instruments inflict structural damage that compromises tooth longevity.

It's remarkable that such respectable studies are mostly ignored by the curriculum writers of modern dentistry.

They continue to instruct dental students on the almost exclusive use of high-speed rotary instruments.

Still, people like Banerjee and Brännström before him continue to haunt the dental profession with the hard light of truth.

Dutch professor Jo Frencken is today one of the top advocates of the Minimally Invasive approach.

He conducted quality studies between 2012 and 2018. Some findings:

1. Microfracture Incidence was less than 5% for ART-treated teeth compared to 72% with drills.
2. Cracks after ART (when present) were superficial (under 50 μm) and non-propagating.
3. ART fillings had an over 85% 10-year survival average compared to under 60% for drill fillings.
4. ART teeth required 80% fewer RCT's over a decade. (Root canals are actually 98% avoidable!)
5. Conclusion: Minimally invasive techniques preserve dentin integrity and reduce long-term failure.

These are serious research findings. The ART method returned vastly superior results on every conceivable measure.

Evidence like this shouts at the inadequacy of mechanical drill and fill methods. It completely validates why most client visits are frightening experiences!

Will dentistry listen? Frencken goes further:

1. Drill shear forces plus heat disrupt dentin's hydroxyapatite-collagen matrix.
2. Cracks propagate along dentinal tubules (like splitting wood grain).
3. ART style hand excavators follow natural caries pathways, avoiding healthy tissue.
4. ART Fillings use chemically bonded glass ionomers that reinforce dentin.
5. Frencken quotes: "Drilling teeth is like repairing a Ming vase with a jackhammer. ART is the conservator's toolkit."

The dental college curriculum is deeply flawed. Unnecessary pain and trauma, plus less healthy! Wrong. ART is a complete game changer.

Rockefeller dentistry might well be a recent iteration which has little semblance to healing at all! I feel like Hegel!

Frencken is a leader in this revival. But there are many others.

You can just ignore it (like they did with mercury amalgam for many years) or you can start to look at safe and effective alternatives right away.

What will the industry do? Will it grudgingly change, or will it happily and eagerly change? Would you care to guess?

Meantimes, one solution appears in the form of holistic, alternative dentists who forsake the drill completely. These are awake dentists working within the industry:

1. The IABDM is the International Academy of Biological Dentistry and Medicine. They are a group of dentists who recognize the risks in many current dental treatments, and who pledge to use only biocompatible materials.
2. IAOMT stands for International Academy of Oral Medicine and Toxicology. They advocate a health-first approach.
3. The HDA is the Holistic Dental Association. It supports dentists who offer non-invasive treatments. They will refer to member dentists.

Ultimately, the only true test is if the dentist is committed to doing an ART-only treatment! This, and only this, is the passing grade for "ancient gold-standard dentistry".

When you find a gold-standard ART-only dentist, you'll surely know that nearly all your oral health issues are in the rear-view.

Regrettably, ART will not replace what's already been irreparably damaged by invasive dentistry. What it will do is ensure that irreparable damage never happens again!

And speaking of absurdity, is there anything more off the wall than three goofballs holding powerful precision instruments?

23
CHAPTER

Conversion

Premise: The Brothers Marx after two years at a dental concentration camp.

Characters: Groucho, Chico, and Harpo.

Setting: A large dining room at a lavish New York dental convention. Brothers seated at a corner table.

Chico: "Eh, you like da diamond bur, using da fine-grit 856-014?"

Groucho: "I only taper with a 330 carbide. (*nods to the adjacent table*) Look out. They're listening."

Chico: "No axial reduction for me. I just do da shoulder margins with 0.5mm chamber and 6° taper. You stupid about dat or what?"

Harpo: (*Honk, honk. Sharp whistle*)

Groucho: "Never mind him, he's shy today. So whadda bout your occlusal clearance, those proximal contacts all right? Mandibular molars are tough business."

A dentist from Spain leans into the conversation.

"Hola, mi nombre es Hidalgo. I do MB2, with #15 K-file and EDTA. And you?"

Chico: "Justa da ProTaper Gold for me. TF Adaptive with da wave irrigation. Apex locator, 20 minute obturation."

Hidalgo: "Ah, cold lateral condensation."

Groucho: "He has no idea what he's talking about. He needs an apical extrusion rate of 30%, otherwise, kaput."

Chico: "Hey, why you wanna kaput me?"

Harpo: (*Toot, toot. Whistle*)

Groucho: "Self-etch, 7th-gen."

Chico: "Naa... Total-etch wit 37% phosphoric, double-layer hydrophobic resin."

Hidalgo: "Hey, you guys do 3 years in dental concentration camp or something?"

Groucho: "It was only 2 years. The company sent us there."

Hidalgo: "Por que?"

Chico: "We weren't upselling to crowns enough."

Hidalgo: "And now you are?"

Groucho: "Top producers".

Hidalgo: "Maybe you not care much for ethic."

Groucho: "Gonna change soon."

Chico: "Incremental curing in 2mm layers. No marginal staining or cusp fractures."

Groucho: "35Ncm torque, Type IV bone."

Hidalgo: "I don't do those."

Chico: "And we gonna stop also."

Hidalgo: "Nice. Why?"

Groucho: " 100% unethical. We can't look ourselves in the mirror anymore."

Hidalgo: "No so healthy, si?"

Groucho: "Total joke. Yet, they still pay."

Hidalgo: "So where you go now?"

Groucho: "We're hearing good things about minimal intervention. Radically different approach to the task."

Chico: "We switch now, full time. MID. Just simple healing."

Hidalgo: "Your company let you?"

Chico: "We quit."

Groucho: "We open our new ART clinic on Monday. "

Hidalgo: "Hey, I like, I like. I join you por favor?"

Groucho: "You wanna join us?"

Hidalgo: "Si. I make big money. But I no like stealing, no mas."

Chico: "HEY! Sit down, Hidalgo! We buy you a drink!"

24

CHAPTER

The *Living Tooth*

Core points:

1. Alkalinity and optimal dental wellness.
2. The layers of the tooth.
3. Does fluoride bring benefits?
4. Dental college ignores the obvious.
5. Why root canals carry high risk.
6. Good teeth are very sexy.

Your teeth deserve to live as long as the rest of your body. It's an outrageous claim, but on Pluto it makes complete sense.

Let's find out what Pluto knows. Dental enamel is primarily calcium (Ca) and phosphate (P, O_4). Combined with the hydroxy base (O, H), and arranged in a unique rod-like lattice framework, it is the strongest material in the body.

It's called a hydroxy-apatite matrix. It loves the alkaline side of the pH scale, and is damaged by the acidic side.

Acids mainly originate from foods (especially the cheap sweet drinks and highly processed foods) and from bacteria (which secrete the acid as a waste product).

These in various combinations result in cavities. Stopping this acidic attack is a key strategy to dental longevity.

Bacteria inhabit dental crevices and "food traps" where they can find sustenance. Excellent oral hygiene flushes them out.

A good dentist will know if you have food traps that may bring future problems.

Inside the outer enamel layer is the dentin. It's softer and is sensitive. It cushions biting pressures.

It can harden into a secondary protective dentin if the enamel is damaged. Enamel is inorganic and cannot regrow.

The innermost layers are where the pulp and nerves are. The capillaries in this layer nourish the tooth, keeping it vital.

Gum health is linked. A holistic dental hygienist is the best bet for coaching on optimal gum wellness. Choose one with a relaxed and communicative approach.

Remineralization is the attempt to bring back an enamel substitute. Since enamel can't regrow, the saliva selectively brings supplemental minerals to plug gaps in demineralized enamel.

Here's where the fluoride question gets interesting. Most think of fluoride as a poison (which it normally is), however, it has a remarkable property of turning demineralized enamel into a new compound called fluoro-apatite.

The hydroxy part of the enamel's hydroxy-apatite matrix is what gets denatured first by acidic attack.

The fluoride can apparently bond with the remaining calcium-phosphorus to form the new fluoro-apatite. It works by swapping ions. It then becomes a catalyst for new stronger dental enamel.

This area deserves serious research. It would confirm that fluoride has a dual nature: very harmful when ingested, yet a restorative catalyst in dentistry.

It has been claimed that new fluoro-apatite is even stronger that original enamel in resisting acidic degradation. That would be remarkable. However, avoiding acidic exposure is always the first thing.

Paracelsus now drops in for a moment: "Ahem… the dose makes the poison."

Wow. He's gone again! That was quick! I think he meant that a poisonous substance can also bring benefits when used in carefully controlled amounts.

Tooth structure

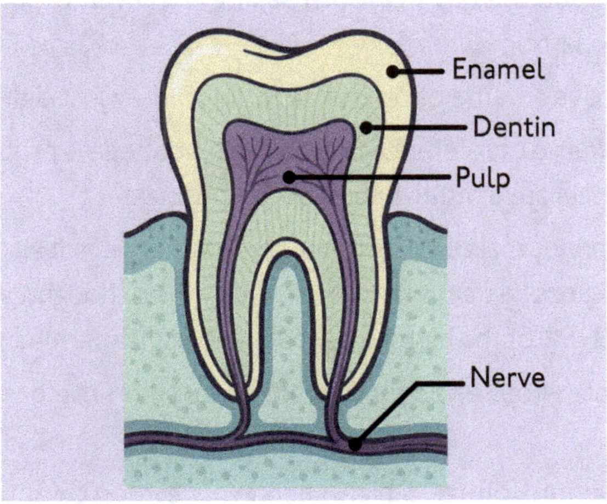

Brushing your teeth with a softer brush reduces the likelihood of gum irritation, which might lead to more serious issues.

Dental colleges are remarkable places. They are often high-security installations, complete with cameras. So, one gains entry by following a student into the attached cafeteria.

We make our way to the second floor, where we spot an amazing poster in the third-year endodontics lab.

It shows the pulp-dentin wall as glass smooth. Students are instructed how to place latex (gutta percha) material (which might or might not have additives) to fill the space inside this wall, for the root canal treatment.

(My estimation is that over 80% of these are avoidable. See chapter 7 I, RCT solutions.)

The only problem with this large poster, is that it's quite false. On the inner walls of the dentin are actually thousands of tiny microtubules, which are the capillaries and nerves that carry nutrients to the dentin-enamel and help it stay strong.

These microtubules have the potential to harbor harmful anaerobic bacteria, which is why root canals should be avoided.

We're puzzled by how these dental college instructors don't know about these thousands of microtubules. Maybe its like the South Sea islanders who couldn't see the large colonial sailing ship even though it was right there in their harbor.

They didn't have a frame of reference for it, so they just didn't see it.

The missing frame of reference for the dental college is probably tied into how root canals are a multi-billion dollar business.

That kind of money makes it hard to see some basic things. It also explains why they don't take ozone treatment very seriously. Even though it's a necessity, as it eliminates 99.9% of the harmful bacteria, and has no harmful side effects.

George Meinig wrote a widely referenced book on the bacterial risks of RCT's.

This is why dental college is high-security. They don't want anyone from the outside world to unexpectedly see their ship of fools, in case they fall overboard.

The teeth are really amazing creations. When they're healthy, it's much more likely the whole body will also be healthy! What a deal!

Taking care of your teeth should be fun. Lets face it, it might be boring. That's why a few good laughs helps everything along.

Teeth are sexy only when they're shiny and well. Otherwise, the person tends to mumble a lot. Not fun.

Come on, have great teeth. You'll thank yourself later. A lot.

You might even become a yogi, living way up on some mountain. People will come to you on pilgrimage, and you'll smile broadly. They'll all say "Wow! That magic yogi has such great teeth!"

You'll look around for a magic yogi, then, finally, you'll realize they're referring to YOU! Wow!

And then you'll tell them all about a great book you read. The somewhat obscure Darles Chickens maritime classic "A Sail of Two Titties".

On a very different front, a most clever undercover investigation took place. Be forewarned. It wasn't pretty at all....

25

CHAPTER

Undercover

Core points:

1. An undercover investigation on dental variability.
2. Dentists often chose treatment plans for the high income.
3. Variability in diagnosis was extreme.
4. A comedic reinterpretation of the investigators' acute bafflement.

Dental healing starts with us. Our good hygiene, good diet, and sensible prevention.

But we do have to visit dentists from time to time, and this can make or break our dental futures.

Variability in dental care is scary!

A 1997 edition of Reader's Digest had a William Ecenbarger article titled "How Honest Are Dentists?".

It was a very frightening article! Ecenbarger went undercover on 50 dentists across the USA. Not only that, but he told them that he had an unlimited insurance plan!

Oh, my goodness. This is like putting a fancy dinner in front of a pack of dogs, and saying "Don't touch this, please!"

He chose dentists at random out of the phone book. He showed each one an x-ray from his "dentist back home", which showed an issue with the #30 tooth, a molar. Otherwise he had no issues.

1. The first dentist said "you need five teeth crowned, including #30, plus additional work." Cost: $6,300."
2. The next dentist said "Five crowns". The teeth needing repairs were different! The cost was $5,200.
3. The third dentist said: "Whoever has been working on your mouth really knows his stuff." No charge.
4. The fourth said "A crown on #30 plus crowns on six others for cosmetic reasons. Ecenbarger apparently stormed out before an estimate was given.
5. The next dentist said "You need 11 crowns, plus other work. It will cost $17,000. Do this and you will have no worries about your teeth for the next 30 years. By the way, you and I are going to become great friends."

At this point, Ecenbarger checked into a Holiday Inn for a week, spending most of his time in the bar, sampling a wide variety of beverages, and listening to salsa song covers by a local band.

Finally he was ready to resume. Somewhat hung over, he was told

6. "$21,000 will bring you up to grade".
7. Next, he got two estimates: "Necessities (4 crowns not including #30): $5,300, and extra cosmetic work: $17,800. Total: $23,100. You may as well get it all done now, since you have the insurance."
8. The next dentist said "Tell me what your insurance limits are, and we'll proceed from there."
9. Next up, he was told he needed a "bare bones" of $10,300, but "ideally", all 28 teeth crowned for only $27,500."

A few days went by as Ecenbarger lost himself in binge eating and medicinal hallucinogens. He emerged to hear:

10. "You need a full-mouth reconstruction, at a cost of $39,500. You'll have the GREATEST SMILE!"
11. Shaken to the core, Ecenbarger was next told: "17 crowns (NOT including #30) for $28,200".

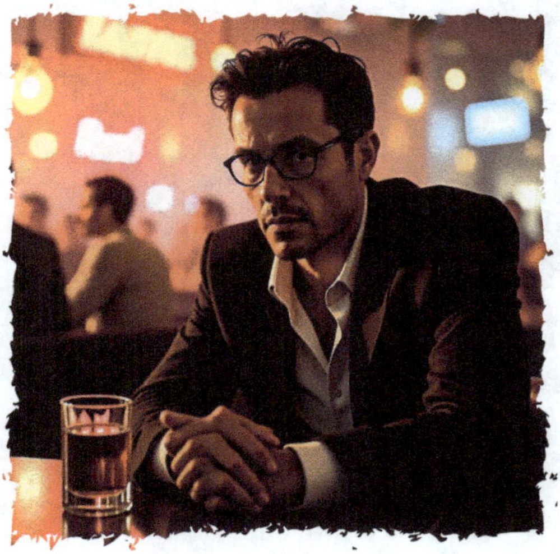

Ecenbarger flew to New York. He sat in jazz clubs and drank a lot. He tried to wrap his mind around it all. If this is journalism, he thought, I need to join a convent. So what with the nun clothing. At least I'll have my teeth!

Then he saw the sign outside the luxurious high-rise.

"I entered an impressive office – handsome furniture, art on the walls, oriental carpets on hardwood floors. Baroque music wafted from invisible speakers. The dentist was a trim, athletic man, and as he examined my teeth, he shook his head in displeasure. Finally, he sighed and invited me to a private conference room. "The news is not good, and you're lucky you have insurance," he said. He handed me a treatment plan that said I needed 21 crowns and veneer on six lower front teeth. Cost: $62,300."

Ecenbarger went directly to a travel agent and purchased a ticket for Kerguelen Island, the most remote place on the planet.

On the way out, he bumped into an expert from a local dental college who said: "Dentistry is an art based on scientific knowledge".

When Ecenbarger's article appeared in the February '97 edition, it was panned by dental authorities for being "mean and cruel".

We step back. We pause, reflect a bit... and we soberly ask: "How could it have come to this?"

A positive upshot to this entire episode is that National Geographic picked up the story, and did a colorful feature on "The penguins, albatrosses, and drunk hermit of Kerguelen Island".

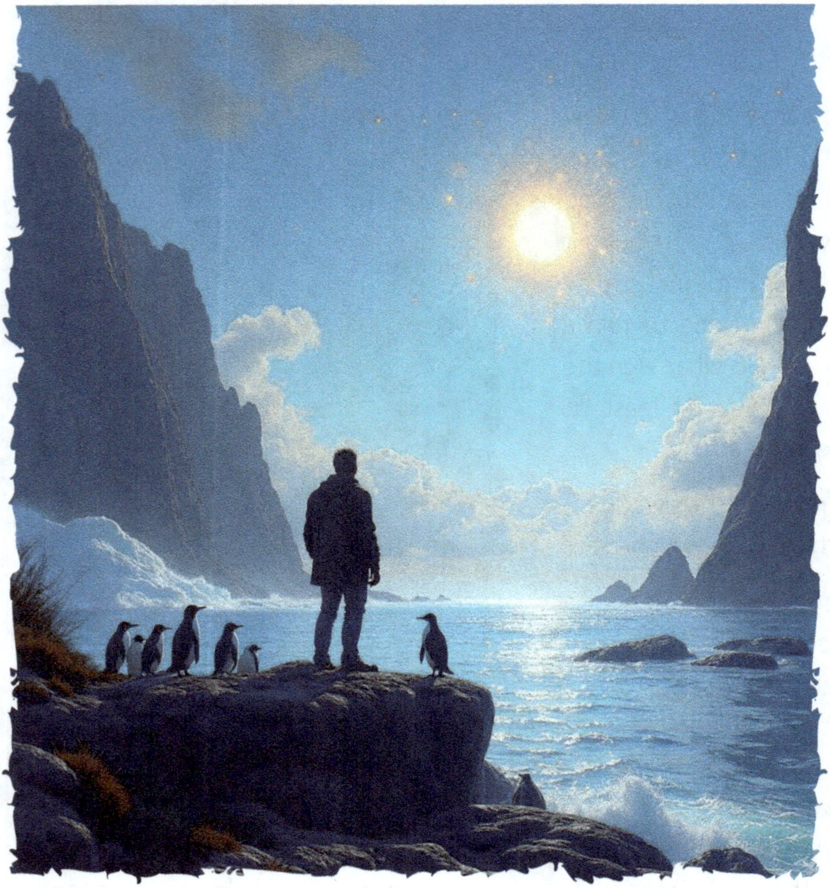

It ran next to a long feature on angry RV-driving pensioners (with small dogs) demanding clothing-optional KOA's while blockading state highways.

Bader and Shugars did an influential 1995 paper on variation in dental treatment diagnoses.

Key points of the paper:

1. Dental decision-making is not purely objective. It is influenced by subjective judgment.
2. A primary driver of the diagnostic variation is "clinical uncertainty", a lack of strong, definitive evidence for the superiority of one treatment approach over another.
3. Long-term health outcomes were not prioritized. The dentists had zero training in "longevity goals".

There's a "call to action" here. This call to action is NOT illicit substances!

It's the need for dental curricula to be trimmed by at least half, and this half replaced with practical healing content. REAL dentistry. Not fake.

The OTHER half of the curriculum needs to be moved to the Economics department where it properly belongs.

Undercover investigations like this tell us things we're apparently "not supposed to know".

[The above account was strongly re-edited for creative purposes but the figures are accurate, accounting for currency valuations.]

Meantime, bare light bulbs buzz and blink unevenly….

26 CHAPTER

Beckett

Title: Waiting for Go.

(A Brief Dramaticule in the Style of Samuel Beckett)

Characters:

V – A haggard patient, slumped in a dental chair.

D – A gloomy dentist, staring at his hands.

(*A single bare bulb flickers. The distant hum of a drill, eternally on the verge of starting.*)

V: (*mumbling, fingers probing cheek*) "…can't go on."

D: (*nods, doesn't look up*) "Must go on."

V: "The drill."

D: (*shrugs*) "The drill."

(*Silence. The bulb buzzes.*)

V: "Heat. Vibration. Micro-fractures. Pulp necrosis. You know."

D: (*wearily picks up a spoon, lets it clatter to the tray*) "Or."

V: "Or?"

D: (*gestures vaguely*) "ART."

V: (*scoffs, then winces*) "Atraumatic."

D: (*nods*) "Win."

V: "Win?"

D: Win. (*pause*) "Less pain."

V: "Less pain."

D: "Better healing."

V: *(long silence)* "...why not?"

D: *(shrugs again, pushes the drill away with his foot)* "Habit."

(The bulb brightens imperceptibly. The drill's hum fades. D lifts the spoon. V opens his mouth. The light holds - then flickers.)

V: *(muffled, around the spoon)* "Is it... working?"

D: *(peering)* "Probably."

V: "That you?"

D: *(pauses)* "Me what?"

(long pause).

V: "Whistling."

D: "Could be."

V: "Is it?"

D: *(a 30 second pause, then...)* "Affirmative."

V: "Oh."

D: "Yep."

V: "First time?"

D: *(Pauses to carefully study his own reflection in the dusty mirror)* "Yep."

(Silence)

(V exhales)

(D reaches for a vial of GIC)

(after one minute)

D: "Finished."

V: "Yeah?"

(a long pause)

V: "Invoice?"

D: "Coming."

V: "When?"

D: "Soon."

V: "Now?"

D: "Relief."

V: "Relief."

D: "ART."

V: "You know."

D: "I know."

(Silence)

(Curtain)

FIN

[editor's note: to further add to the irony, one realizes that one of the stars of this skit was .. the bulb…]

27

CHAPTER

Clarity

Core points:

1. How and why dentists leverage authority.
2. How to spot deceptions.
3. Ensuring you get the treatment you actually need.
4. Why saving a tooth is the best possible investment.

"I completely disagree with your diagnosis of the root canal procedure."

"Why?"

"Kills the tooth."

"Accepted standard of care."

"Not my standard at all."

This might be a typical conversation. A living tooth might last a lifetime. A root canal is a done deal.

Dentists leverage "authority bias" to make educated guesses seem like certainties. Is it intimidation? It always happens.

Here are some "four alarm fire" diagnoses, and the correct relaxed responses:

1. The Imminent tooth danger scare: "This tooth needs a crown, root canal etc". (insert expensive, irreversible treatment here).

   Unspell. Relax, get a second opinion, especially one that explains how to save the tooth with MID. All teeth can be saved. Never give up on a tooth. Ever.

2. The mystery "micro-leakage" diagnosis: "This filling needs to be replaced. You need a total makeover, etc". Relax. Ply him with tooth longevity objectives.
3. Overdiagnosing gum disease: "You need a $1,200 deep cleaning." Relax. "Have you tried holistic methods?"
4. The phantom cracked tooth: "I see a hairline crack. You need a crown!" Relax. "Is it causing symptoms? Is it really a crack? Do you have a boat payment due?"
5. The bone loss boogeyman: "I see severe issues on this x-ray!" Relax. "Bone density naturally varies"
6. The You Grind upsell: "You need an $800 night guard!" Relax. "I have zero symptoms. Could you show me the wear patterns?"
7. The cosmetic perfection trap: "Your fillings look old/discolored. I need to replace them!" Relax. "Are the restorations functional? Then they're fine."
8. The "preventive" root canal: "This tooth might die someday. We should do a root canal now!" Relax. "Even pulpitis can heal over time."
9. The implant upsell: "This missing tooth will cause untold problems!" Relax. "No it won't."
10. The TMJ Misdiagnosis: "Your pain is caused by "TMJ"; we need a $2,000 splint." Relax. "Stress management, good exercise, etc, cure so many things."

Always:

1. Ask for evidence
2. Request alternatives
3. Delay decisions on hugely expensive/invasive treatments.
4. Trust how you actually feel.

Frank Jerome reminds us: "90% of dental diagnoses are optional and negotiable."

Once you jump, there's no going back. And it isn't just treatment, it's almost always "surgery".

Keeping a healthy oral bioflora and a good pH balance is important prevention. So is cutting out refined sugar completely.

Refined sugar is only a drug. And it's in a majority of highly processed foods. No one knows why, but they sneak it in there.

Become a no sugar person. You don't need it. It stimulates an area of the tongue and it's a drug. Brush well and floss well.

Saving a tooth might require a very aggressive healing protocol (ART along with ozone therapy), but it can very often be accomplished.

Remarkable options exist for saving teeth. Even very damaged teeth can become functional again.

We never allow urgent invasive treatment plans to affect us in the slightest. Dental longevity is our only reality. So is ART.

28

CHAPTER

Zero-Con

Core points:

1. Encountering a persistent con artist.
2. The deceptive upsells of dentistry.
3. Pressure as an indicator of suspect motives.
4. Understanding why dentists try to max their practice profits.

"I have to call a locksmith to open my car! I left my keys locked inside!"

The man in a crumpled suit was urgently asking me for $20, late in the evening at a Los Angeles bus stop. It's always urgent. Always.

LA seems full of either working actors, or wannabe/ looking for work actors. And it's occurred to me: who would make a better con artist than an unemployed actor?

So there I am, being asked for a fresh 20, and he needs it yesterday. I was wearing my casual tan slacks, a nice turquoise cotton shirt, and canvas sneakers.

I tried to ignore him, and finally the bus came and I got on. What did I see after sitting down, but the same guy! He'd boarded the bus. Even though his "apparent car" was still back there.

He resumed plying me for the 20 dollars! I started to get seriously impatient at that point. I pondered physical violence.

So he got the idea, and wandered down the bus, and apparently got at least 10 dollars from someone else!

This is just to illustrate that a serious con artist can be really persistent.

Your teeth want to be well, and they don't want to fall prey to con artists either.

I'm not suggesting here that healthcare professionals who routinely "upsell" are con artists. But skill and persuasion are definitely part of the equation.

Some of those treatments are tremendously lucrative. How lucrative?

Aggressive upselling can increase a dentist's revenue by 50% or even much more, depending on the practice's ethical boundaries and patient demographics.

1. Corporate dental chains often incentivize production quotas, leading to 30 to 50% higher revenue per patient.
2. Unnecessary crowns could produce $800 to $1,500 each vs. $150 to $300 for a filling.
3. Gum issues could lead to $200 to $400 cleanings vs. $50 to $100 preventive visits.
4. Night guards are "high-margin" ($500–$1,500).
5. Porcelain crowns costing the dentist $100 to $300 might sell for $800 to $1,500, for a profit margin of 400–800%.
6. Deep cleaning: dentist cost of $50 to $150 might sell for $300 to $600. Profit margin = 300–500%.
7. Veneers (per tooth), dentist cost = $200 to $500. Sell for $1,000 to $2,500. Profit margin = 400–900%.
8. Invisalign, dentist cost = $500–$1,000, sell for $3,000–$8,000. Profit margin = 500– 1,000%.

These are estimates. Some dentists prioritize procedures that insurers reimburse well for. Example: crowns over fillings.

A patient needing 1 or 2 fillings ($300 to $600) might be upsold 2 crowns ($1,600 to $3,000). Cost = 5x.

The thing I've learned from con artists is that there is always pressure. No pressure = much less likely to be a con.

Don Corleone once growled (swishing an amaretto, cotton pads stuffed in downturned mouth):

"And you come here on the day of my daughter's wedding… to ask me for permission to undercut my business?"

Never be conned into thinking that "dental experts" know more about your teeth than you do.

Dental healing is a high art form. But not everyone appreciates certain artists. The hand tools only approach of ART is a fabulous starting point.

Before I had my EXCELLENT hand tool ART restoration, I was quoted by several dentists (who took either a cursory look or a visual exam and X-ray) that it was a root canal situation. WRONG.

And yet, they pushed it because it's the easy road for them. As one president would say: Sad!

We never fall for cons, and we never let ourselves be pressured into expensive treatments. Ones we know nothing about! Simplicity is always best.

29

CHAPTER

Resist

Core points:

1. A dental whistleblower reveals key inside secrets.
2. Dental profit motivation colliding with client need.
3. The upsell culture revealed.
4. Acute discernment is essential.

Walking the dusty streets of Los Algodones, Mexico, you might hear a hundred serious remarks like "root canal and crown". You're looking for ART only treatment, and every dentist there is revving their high-speed handpieces.

You'll hear constant sales pitches for implants. This is about as far from ART as it gets, so there's no need to go into detail on it. Suffice it to say that a certain segment of the market wants this.

I'm not here to argue against what some people really want. Many get sold on "complete smile makeovers". For me that's as far as it gets from any kind of healing. So I'm just not going there.

Let's now shift the scene to a large North American clinic, where a working dentist was expelled from a large practice because her style of dentistry wasn't meeting "quotas". This is a view from the inside:

1. "You trust your dentist to tell you what you need to know, so that you can weigh your options. That's fine if the dentist is completely impartial about selling care to an unsuspecting public.

2. Over the years, dentists have received training from practice management firms and product manufacturers on how to sell more dentistry, sell treatment plans, and convince clients to commit to expensive lucrative treatment.
3. They say "It's all OK since the patients need to get work done anyway, so why not sell patients on the most expensive treatment that you can."
4. It doesn't seem to matter if the treatments are more invasive than necessary, they are convinced that it is justified because it is how lots of other dentists practice. It is 'within the standard of care'.
5. I was fired from an office where I worked because they said I wasn't producing enough crowns. They said I was using burrs that are too small and not cutting away enough tooth structure, and I should do dentistry the way the owner's boss did.
6. Since each dentist has their own license that they are responsible for, I knew I had a right to practice according to how I was trained and my philosophy. So I told them that if they wanted me to do more crowns, then they should have the front office schedulers schedule more people for me that NEED crowns.
7. For stable revenue, they just wanted me to cut some number of crowns per month whether I thought it was a necessary treatment or not. They did a lot of crowns at that office!
8. That is the current culture in most dental offices. In some offices, the entire staff makes bonuses based on the money collected. So everyone is so nice to you, and tells you how great veneers will look. Or how great implants are and how bad partials are (they cost MUCH less by the way). Implants are a big money maker.
9. This is all justified in their minds by the fact that you might actually need some dental care, so they 'up sell' and use fear and vanity to motivate you. They will tell you things are urgent, and the awful things that will happen if you don't hurry up and get the treatment that the doctor has recommended for you.
10. They will often have the dental hygienist repeat it, and the assistants as well. This is done to reinforce the truthfulness effect. If you've heard

it several times, "it must be true"... If you go for a second opinion, you are likely to land in a similar situation, but they might trash the other dentist's treatment plan to get you to come to them for treatment. I've seen this happen!

11. A true second opinion should be by someone with other options available. Take your time and get as many alternate views as you want. Any dentist that discourages this can be considered unprofessional.
12. Even if you decide not to get care in a holistic office, I highly recommend seeking an opinion from such a dentist. They usually are lower key about telling you whatever you want to know and are usually more at ease about you taking your time making a decision.
13. They usually will not act insulted or hurt if you choose to get the treatment elsewhere. It is your choice and the holistic community as a whole really gets this concept of freedom of choice and sovereignty over your body and your health."

This describes dentistry's worst face. How much of the dental industry does this account represent? A little or a lot?

Viable living tissue is lost that cannot be replaced. It's a permanent injury. There's no going back after that invasive treatment.

The recommended lucrative treatments are urgent! They always are!

This type of dental practice is known as a "crown mill". They upsell. There have been high profile class action lawsuits about these types of chains.

You know about ART now, so you know the for-real dental healing path. You know what dental longevity is!

This is how dentistry is supposed to be! You're never going back to that old injurious way - ever!

You're on the path to glory!

30

CHAPTER

Healing Hygiene

Core points:

1. Where do we find dental healers?
2. Dental hygienists are uniquely positioned.
3. Summarizing what hygienists do.
4. A.R.T. as the logical on-ramp for the best dentalcare.

In Mexico, the traditional healers are known as curanderos. Most are found in the smaller villages. They use plants, roots and ancient methods.

During travels, I would receive warnings that those remote areas are sometimes dangerous. Very sobering.

Still, we need to understand the healer's methods. They can add tremendous value to our dental healing.

The ultimate foundation for healing has to be Light. It's the substrate of all things, at least according to quantum science.

In this measure, quanta, light, and energy are interlinked. Sunshine is the essential ingredient.

In terms of practitioners, a good holistic-minded dental hygienist is excellently positioned to provide good long-term dental healing.

We ensure that we can converse with them comfortably. They won't be trained in the various invasive procedures of dentists.

Might some hygienists be acting as "on-ramps" for invasive dentistry? Hopefully not!

The dental hygiene program taught in the colleges must not just be a "de-fanged" dental program. It has to be healing-based in its own right.

The number one value of a dental hygienist would be their ability to do ART restorations. Their highest calling!

I've sought out this capability in the dental hygienists, and made remarkable progress.

According to their course curriculum, hygienists are trained in:

1. Dental care but not in surgery. A huge plus.
2. Oral anatomy and physiology.
3. Nerve pathways (trigeminal nerve) and occlusion (bite alignment).
4. Diagnosis of gum problems.
5. Ability to do scaling and planing.
6. All diagnoses including x-rays.
7. Applying dental sealants.
8. Client consultations on effective prevention practices.
9. Soft-tissue management (gingival massage, laser therapy).
10. Sterilization management.
11. Administering all anesthetics. (Non-contamination is a must.)
12. Patient assessment.
13. Outreach programs in the community.

Licensed hygienists are well skilled. But are they licensed to do ART? Will hygienists be true curanderos?

We have naturopathic doctors. Now we need naturopathic dental healers. Urgently!

Maybe you will be encouraged to go into serious dental healing yourself. Perhaps you'd choose to take the route of dental hygiene.

Or perhaps you'd go into regular dentistry with a strong healer's mindset, like many have. Where you'd be up against an industry that doesn't comprehend a thing you're doing!

Either way, the rewards could be amazing. Crush it!

In the meantime, a London flat is the scene of a healing procedure that, if more widely known, would spare people considerable trauma and pain…

31

CHAPTER

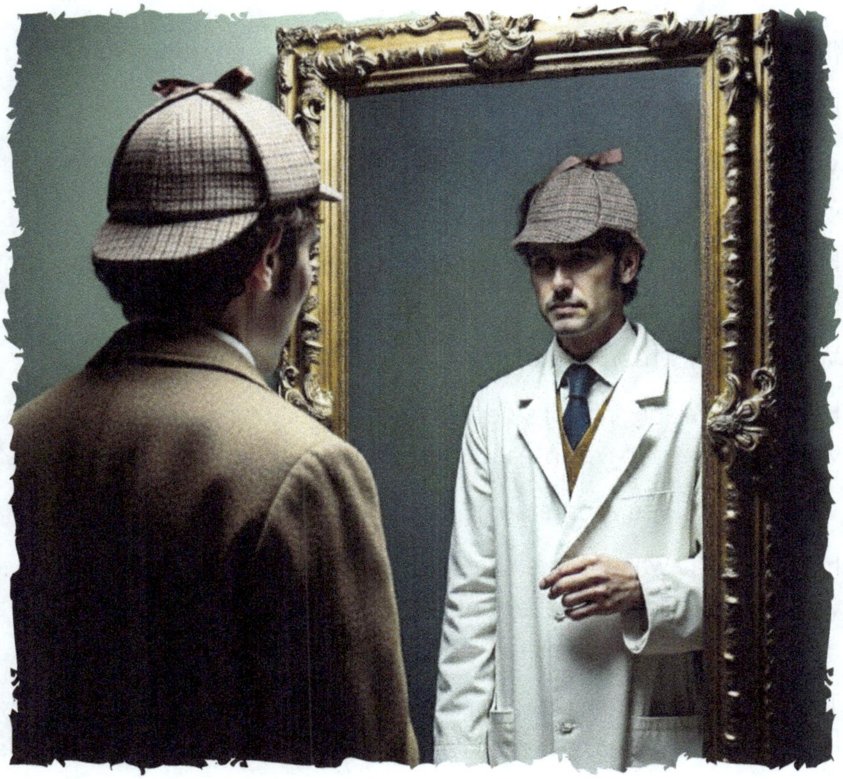

Holmes 1

Scene: 221B Baker Street, the new location of the Sherlock Holmes Dental Spa.

Sunlight streams through tall windows. There are trays of small hand excavators, mixing pads for glass ionomer cement, CR gel vials. Holmes examines a patient's tooth under a focused light magnifier. Watson assists, handing him a tiny spoon-shaped instrument. A nervous young Mr. Dobbs sits in the chair.

Holmes: (*voice precise*) "Watson, this is a clear indicator for ART. A demineralization zone on the distal surface. Entirely within the dentin, the enamel above is intact. No need for turbines here." (He uses the spoon instrument expertly)

"Mr. Dobbs, you will feel perhaps a slight scraping sensation. No more."

Dobbs: "No needle? No drill?"

Watson: (*warmly*) "None whatsoever, Mr. Dobbs. Holmes' methods are about minimal intervention.

Holmes: (*working with precision*) "Precisely, Watson. However, let us not overlook the real benefit - saving lives."

Watson: "Say what, Holmes?"

Holmes: "Watson, injurious dentistry leads to suffering. That much is obvious. However, it may also lead to other complications. Rather serious ones."

Watson: "Ah, I see your reasoning, Holmes."

Holmes: "And what's more, Watson, is that the profession doesn't take it very seriously! In fact, we're about to get proof on our doorstep in just a moment, if I'm not mistaken."

The door bursts open. Dr. Salazar Stevens stands framed in the doorway. He is large, red-faced, dressed in a heavy, old-fashioned dental apron. He carries a bulky, gleaming engine drill case.

Stevens: (*booming voice*) "Holmes! Where is your standard of care!"

Holmes doesn't flinch, finishing the placement of Fuji IX with a final touch.

Holmes: (*calmly, not turning*) "Stevens. Your timing, as ever, is intrusive. I'm preventing a situation of guaranteed suffering."

Stevens: (*slams his drill case onto a side table with a thud.*) "Ceasing suffering? Pah! The standard way is the only way! You must drill deeply to remove everything!"

Holmes: "And inject for pain control?"

Stevens: "Of course!"

Holmes: "You're quite mistaken, Stevens. Your undercut methods and sedated overtreatments cause loss of living viable tissue. A very serious negligence."

Stevens: "Be careful, Holmes. I shall have you for slander."

Holmes: "And I shall have you for assault, Stevens. Are you almost finished?"

Watson: (*stepping forward impatiently*) "Dr. Stevens! Holmes' method is not poisonous"

Stevens: "Oh! You refer to mercury. We have been phasing it out."

Watson: "Phasing out is not realistic, Stevens. Neither is inducing fear."

Stevens: "Bah! We don't induce fear!"

Holmes: (*looking up*) "Then how many of your clients actually enjoy visiting you for treatment, Stevens?"

Stevens: "You're being ridiculous, Holmes. Dentistry was never meant to be FUN!"

Holmes: "Except here, Stevens."

Dobbs: (*facing Stevens*) "He's right, Sir. This didn't hurt at all. In fact, it was most pleasant."

Watson: (*heaves a big sigh*) "Have you seen enough, Stevens?"

Holmes: "Stevens, your drills weaken teeth, resulting in fracture. The focused heat results in pulp trauma. Your large preparations necessitate more invasive future repairs. It is a cycle of disintegration. And... for what?"

Stevens: "HA! Next, you'll tell me that you're aiming for dental longevity!"

Holmes looks at Watson and shrugs. Then they look at Stevens, who appears to be frozen on the spot. Stevens tries to utter a reply, but can't.

Holmes: "My word. A stress seizure! Watson, could you call Mrs. Hudson? I believe our visitor has encountered reality in a most jarring fashion! A good cup of hot tea will let him regain his senses."

Soon, Mrs. Hudson leads a shocked Stevens down the stairs.

Holmes: (turning to the others) "And for ourselves, I believe a good hot tea will also do us all very well. Please do join us, Dobbs. I'm so glad to hear that you had such a positive experience at the… healer."

32

CHAPTER

Apprentice

Core points:

1. How tutors expedite the learning process.
2. Circumventing the cost and wait times for important coursework.

I was convinced. I was also impatient. I had to learn how to do a hands-on dental restoration.

Then I remembered.

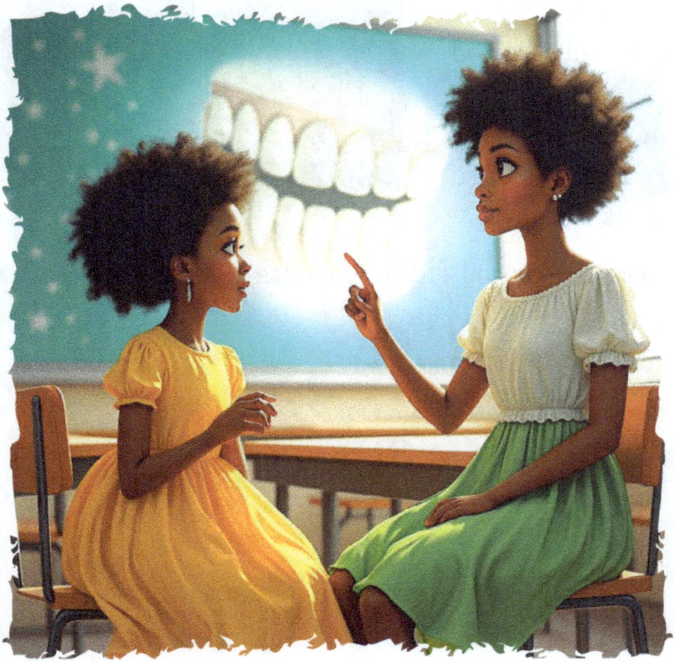

When I was 20, I really wanted to learn to drive a truck. However I hadn't set aside much money for the two-month truck driver course.

So I looked in the paper (all the ads were in the back of the newspaper in those days), to the "work wanted" section. Sure enough, I found several licensed truck drivers looking for work. I called a couple of them.

One fine trucker was available that very day. I went out to meet him. I explained my situation.

"Will you tutor me on how to drive a truck? I'll pay you by the hour."

The upshot is that within two weeks I had my truck license. A beautiful Class I, along with an air brake endorsement that I'd gotten from a one-day course earlier.

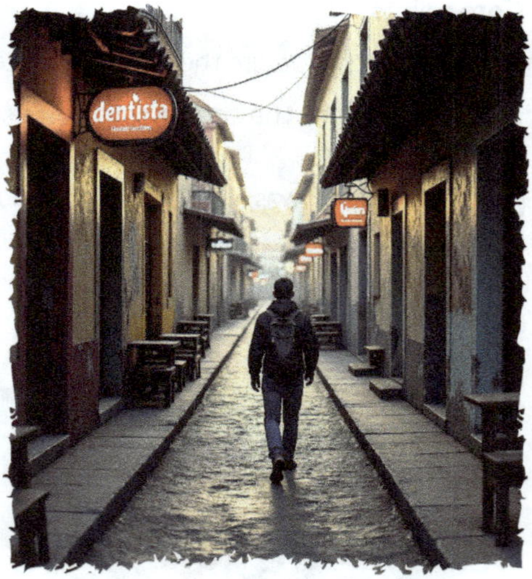

The moral of the story? If you can't find a course, don't worry. Go out and find a tutor. Learn now.

How does this apply to dentistry? Well, I really wanted to learn the ART protocol. However, the course in Canada is only open to certified dental hygienists.

Meaning I'd need to fly to India to find a course that I could take as a normal citizen.

I found a better way. A much better way...

33

CHAPTER

A Lesson

Core points:

1. A disruptive account of being tutored in dental restorations.
2. Treatment providers should innovate for best results..
3. Enriching yourself by acquiring a much needed skill.

Walking the small streets of Los Algodones, Mexico, on the border with Arizona, just choked with literally hundreds of dental clinics, I had an idea. I'd been regrouping to the only espresso cafe, to plot my next moves.

I hadn't yet found a willing dentist to do an ART-only treatment. Still tal-king, still asking. So why not use the time well?

I decided to ask for a basic lesson in restorative technique. I soon found a dentist willing to give me a two hour tutoring session for 100 dollars. Many of these dentists are working intermittently. She was happy to oblige.

I asked her what tools I needed. I went to the local dental supply shop that afternoon (yes, Los Algodones has two of these suppliers) and pic-ked up what I needed.

First, a good typodont. This is a set of plastic teeth to practice on. I bought the child model because it cost 20 dollars only, half the price of the adult model.

I picked up some restoration composite. I already had some hand tools. I bought etcher acid and some adhesive.

The next morning I showed up at her clinic very eager to go. For two hours she watched carefully as I did a few really good looking restorations on those plastic teeth.

I was careful to apply the composite in thin 2 millimeter increments, light curing each layer for 20 seconds.

When it was over, I felt I had turned a new chapter. I was elated. I handed over the 100 dollars with great appreciation.

Doing a good dental restoration is like learning to ride a bike. Once you get it, you're a top-secret dentist.

Would you really need to take a four year degree to learn this? Two weeks is nicer. Or two hours!

Here's the funny thing. The dental profession is probably terrified of the possibility of the public learning to do their own dentistry. Their worst nightmare!

And we don't wish nightmares on anyone. So we keep it secret.

The best thing about learning ART-style restorations is that you're not learning how to use a drill, because that's exactly what you're getting away from.

The authorities shouldn't have a problem if you learn how to do a basic dental restoration. After all, it comes under the heading of self care. Still, it's probably the last thing they wish to contemplate! Ka-ching...!

(This is Chinese for the sound of an old fashioned cash register, before plastic cards. It's also a lovely lake north of Xian.)

If Chinese hobbits were going to treat others and weren't discreet about it, then yes, they would run into problems. The nasties would nail them for being unlicensed.

Regardless, there's probably a great learning experience in getting a typodont and some basic tools. Practice until you feel confident. Watch online videos for guidance.

And yes, find a good tutor. A third year dental college student could be the best choice. This aspiring dentist will have already had multiple training sessions on typodonts, and possibly clinical practice on people as well.

By fourth year, all dental students will have worked with actual patients.

Tutors are usually very affordable. Try offering 40 or 50 dollars per hour. Try offering 10!

And if you want to go first class, then book a working vacation. Find a small Asian country that will let you take the full-fledged ART course. It's usually only one week long. It might turn out to be the best travel you've ever done.

A practical skill like ART might see you through many needs. It's so functional and sensible. You might well want to become a healer-hygienist!

And yes, give your child a typodont at Christmas! That's how geniuses get started! Imagine play-times after that!

[Disclaimer: For general stress-reduction, let only close associates know you have learned this valuable skill.]

34 CHAPTER

Affirm!

Core points:

1. Affirming leads to desired outcomes.
2. Dental health benefits from clear intentions.

Our dental healing journey is not done in a vacuum. We're surrounded by multitudinous narratives.

Some people complain of a discomforting "internal conversation". They mistakenly believe that this is coming from themselves. It is not!

It's part of an energetic flux having its location in the various energy fields surrounding us at any given time. It's coming from a stratum of that field known as the mind or language plane.

There are also other planes. We have a feeling plane. And of course, we have the physical plane!

We have the lottery winner plane, where instant millionaires cannot possibly decide what to buy first!

Dental healing benefits from good affirmative statements that counteract the difficult effects of the ambient noise of the language plane.

Affirmations reorder and restructure these "internal conversations"! Affirmations make our intentions positive!

They are statements that form new structures in the invisible world. They may seem outrageous at times, but that's not the point! The point is that they open up a new field of possibilities!

We need to introduce some good dental healing affirmations. Here are some samples:

1. Excellent dental health is my birthright, and I claim it with joy.

2. My dentist is now the helper of my dental longevity because I know exactly what I'm looking for.
3. My teeth are my friends; where they go, I go, and I only give them the very best.
4. My teeth are alive and well, and I highly value them! It is good!
5. I am a Golden Being of Light, and I spread joy and happiness wherever I go. And my teeth fully agree!
6. I forgive the dentist for having placed very toxic substances like mercury, and for having undercut healthy tissue. He was simply following a very incomplete teaching. Now he knows much better. I'm grateful!
7. My teeth are now becoming the best they can be.
8. I forgive my dentist for having to take a curriculum that did not encourage dental longevity.
9. My teeth are golden prisms of Light; they radiate the fullness of the Glory.
10. My dental treatments are now colored with the golden light of wise understanding.
11. My teeth serve me well because I serve my teeth well.
12. My teeth are healing and becoming stronger because I know the path to their optimal wellness.
13. My chompers shall prosper, and no, that's not bonkers.
14. The rules on optimal dental wellness are simple, sure, and true, and I am understanding these rules better day by day.
15. Dental health is in my future. I'm happy.

These affirmations are spoken out loud, with a purpose.

We get to try out the affirmations that resonate best with us. If it doesn't resonate, we switch to one that does!

When we start to restructure that invisible world, we become masters of our destiny.

It's a pretty good destiny when these forces line up and cohere. Dental healing is a knowing.

35

CHAPTER

S Study

Core points:

1. In Brazil, A.R.T. was tested for public dentistry.
2. Results were legendary.
3. Pulp capping allows biocompatible protection of inner tissues.

There is a pop song that goes:

"When my baby smiles at me,
I go to Rio.
De Janeiro.
I go wild and then,
I have to do the samba,
And la bamba…"

This public service announcement is to suggest that this could be exceedingly expensive, hence, unsustainable.

The trip will set you back several thousand, including the stay-over. You may get to do some samba, watch songwriters pen classic tunes about Ipanema girls waking by, but still….

And when you return, she's so happy to see you and smiles once more… the same all over again?

Much wiser is that when she smiles at you, simply go to the local Whole Foods. There, you may find good quality dental floss, plus other fine condiments such as coconut oil and baking soda, with which to make your own very high-quality dentifrice (see Chapter 55 of this volume).

You will save a fortune, plus you'll have serious dental healing goods.

In Brazil, there is a large statue of Yeshua the timeless healer, on top of a mountain. Below, the beaches of Copacabana bump to the smooth and silky beat of bossanova.

A Brazilian dental researcher named Souza conducted a set of studies on the efficacy of ART for deep caries. The kind that would in 99% of regular cases be diagnosed as a root canal treatment.

This was a large-scale public health initiative done partly to serve those many people who could not afford regular dental treatment.

And also to study the effectiveness of ART treatments in a very broad, well-monitored way.

In all instances, the ART method of conservative treatment was followed. Removing only soft decayed tissue and leaving viable solid tissue, even if discolored. This ART protocol resulted in nearly 100% restoration success.

The testing was done over a 10-year span. This type of investigation has very high accuracy.

If decay is deeper than the dentin layer, it can still be saved. If pulp and nerve are affected, then a person will either feel consistent pain (requiring attention) or a kind of low-key situation where the body's own numbing action has taken over. The body does have a numbing action.

Some people will even numb the pain and carry on because they're too afraid of dentists. That's a sad situation all right. Get treatment right away, but make sure it's the right kind of treatment.

Deep caries can be treated without killing the tooth. Dentists are so quick to give up on problem teeth. If decay has reached the pulp, they won't think twice. Root canal every time.

ART dictates that you leave partly decayed dentin that is structurally sound. Then the body will take care of it from the inside. The Huth study has proven this is the correct way.

GIC acts as a pulp cap. It's biomimetic. It acts as a shield but also helps to build up the tissue so it can turn into secondary dentin.

Secondary dentin is the durable layer that the body will form once the decay is properly removed. Yes, the body will find a way to heal the damage from the inside.

These are hugely important nuances that dentistry totally misses. How many expensive endodontal procedures have been done, which kill the tooth and leave it there as a bacteria-attracting prosthetic? When a bit of creative thinking would have totally saved the tooth.

And truly, you might even end up with a very long living tooth. And that is REAL dentistry.

The Souza study proved that success rates using ART are many times greater than by using the traditional invasive drill method.

Refrigerator magnet note: "Raising the dead is fine, but let's start by raising the living first."

A compelling irony of the 10-year Souza study was that all the people on modest incomes who qualified for this ART treatment ended up with vastly superior results. Compared to the wealthier folks who had regular dentistry for their treatments.

The results speak for themselves. There is simply no denying it. And this is VERY good news!

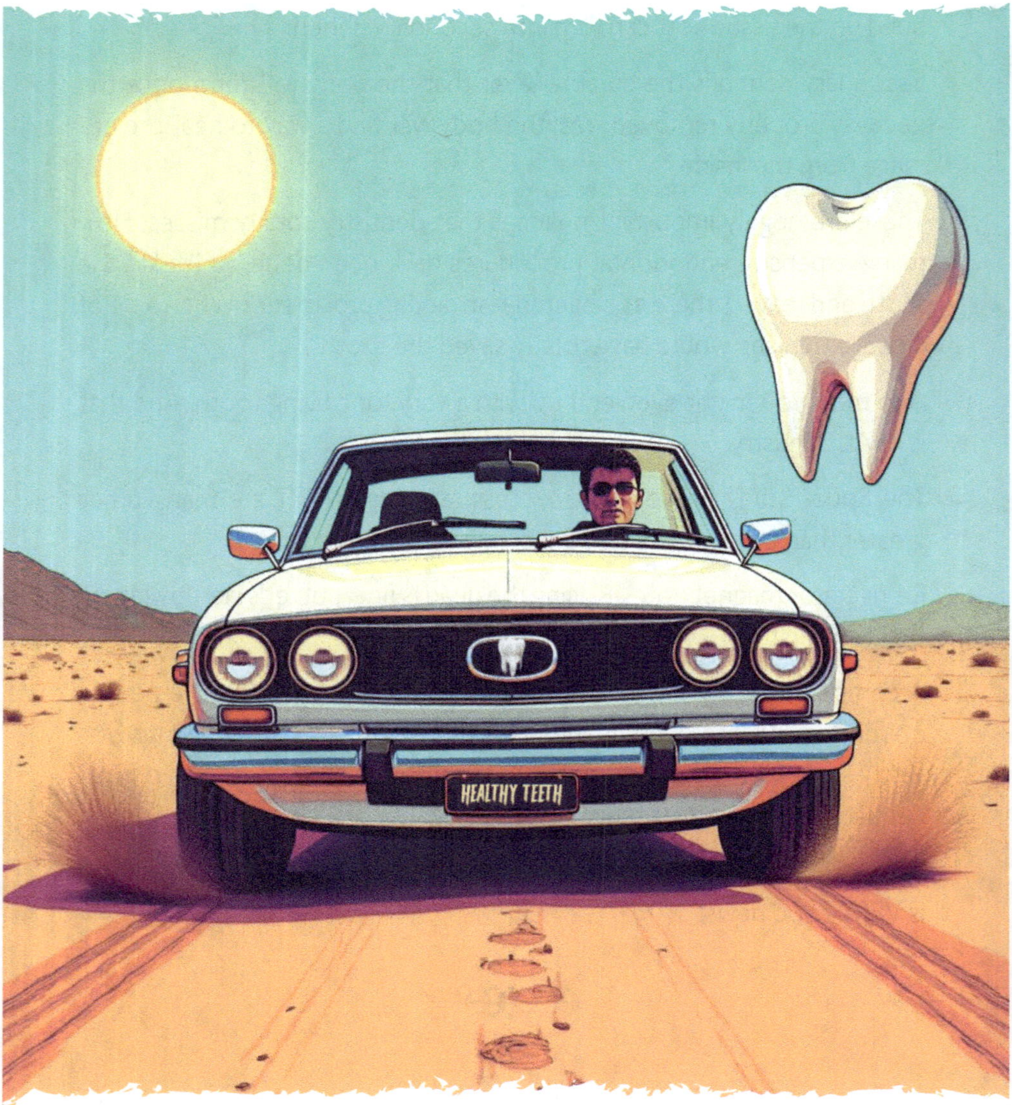
HEALTHY TEETH

36 CHAPTER

MID

Core points:

1. One dental student rebelled against an absurd curriculum.
2. He decided to practice minimalist dentistry on his own terms.
3. Becoming a wandering dental wizard might be feasible.

"This '25 Nissan Versa has only 300 miles on it. It's basically new. You want it?"

The car-hire agent in San Antonio, Texas was showing me one of his available rental cars.

"Sure, why not..." I said, feigning casualness.

The mission? Go find one of the pioneers of the MID (minimally invasive dental) movement. His name is Tim Rainey and his clinic is in a small village in south Texas called Refugio.

This doesn't keep people from flying in from all over North America to have a treatment from him. He's also booked solid for three months.

Rainey is in my opinion a veritable quote machine. Here are a few of my favorites:

1. Asked where he learned his approach to Minimally Invasive Dentistry, Rainey says: "Absolutely not in dental school, that's for certain. From the very first moment in dental school where they showed us a video and said, "Take a high speed drill and do this", I went into full-blown rebellion. It wasn't logical and it didn't make any sense. You couldn't convince me that it was good for the patient or good for the tooth."

2. "With the right kind of prevention, 80% of all dental repair work can be avoided. Most dental work done today is about repairing previous dental work! Yes, 80%!"
3. "Dental decay is primarily driven by the symbiotic relationship between bacteria and acidity, which creates a pathogenic bioflora in your mouth. So raise the pH with alkalinity."
4. "Besides being incredibly poisonous, mercury-amalgam also promotes almost certain cracking of teeth because of the weakening process. You end up with a whole series of iatrogenic (dentistry-caused) disasters."
5. "It's absolutely useless to try to sell (the healthiest products) to dentists. You can't sell them. There are only about five percent of the dentists out there who are out on the cutting edge that have anything. The rest of them finally get in line whenever they feel threatened within their practice. The only way (the healthiest methods will be implemented) is when people say 'I want this for me. I want this for my child. I want to find a dentist who is willing to provide this service.' That's the bottom line."
6. "When they first developed the sodium bicarbonate (baking soda) prophylaxis air abrasion unit, the one that we use for polishing teeth, one of the first things they noticed was how it suppressed pathogenic microbial flora for up to three months."

Rainey is refreshing when he does the straight talk about the dental industry. He should know because he's on the inside!

It was unfortunate that Rainey was booked solid for the next four months! I hadn't made an appointment and I didn't want to force my way into someone else's spot. So I had to move along.

The Nissan made for a great long drive. I returned it to fly over to Monterrey, Mexico, where I looked for ART-trained dentists for five days. Then onto Tijuana for more of the same. Finally, Los Algodones, where I finally found my first ART treatment. At last!

Was it worth all the travel and expense? In a way, yes. Because I wasn't going to give up until I found what I needed. And yes, it was that hard to find a hand-tools-only treatment. This should serve as a sobering heads-up to all those seeking ART.

Obviously you will need to do a lot of prior research before you go fly anywhere looking for ART treatment.

I don't really mind traveling, but I admit this was a bit much. However, having had the PERFECT treatment, I can now say that no effort is too much to obtain what you totally need.

A camperized mini-van with ART tools in the back, next to a full stretch-out bunk, would make you a traveling wizard ART-ist!

Like the bards of old, you'd wander around curing stuff! It could actually be a certified mobile ART clinic.

Currently there are many mobile dental hygienists, so this notion is very close to being reality! Just add ART to hygienist and you're there!

MID is a true dentistry that comes very close to what ART is. The Minimally Invasive philosophy is to preserve vital dental tissue and promote healing.

This is the way dentistry is supposed to be. The ART protocol takes it all the way to the ancient gold-standard. It's literally the best of the best!

Tim Rainey does represent the under 5% or so of dentists who instinctively know that regular dentistry is fundamentally unhealthy.

There are some very conscientious dentists but they seem to be in the under 5% range. They seek ways to do less harm and to cause as little damage as possible.

They are the most ideal candidates to usher in the use of ART in the most mainstream way possible.

All litigation is problematic. But when it's a set-up in advance, we have some serious doo-doo.

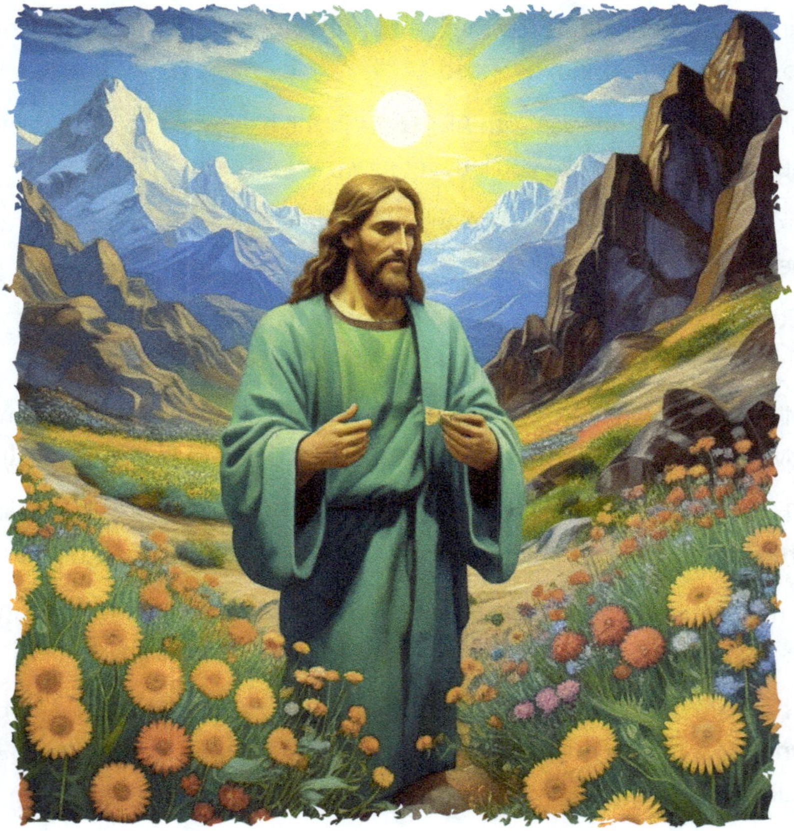

37

CHAPTER

The Curtain

Core points:

1. Powerful healers often find themselves in danger.
2. Powerful forces oppose the craft of healing.
3. Healing is an adjunct to wisdom.

"Do you find issue with this Man? I certainly don't."

Thus asked Pontius Pilate, when he pulled the greatest Healer in the history of civilization in front of a bewildered crowd.

The key was the "important folks" lurking behind. These folks were the industry leaders. We know this because Pilate was the head of state in this Rome-controlled province. Industry leaders tend to congregate near heads of state.

In front of them stood the genuine King! Jesus was the direct lineage heir to the David-Solomon throne of Judea.

Of course. Rome didn't want the real king. So they needed to hold a kangaroo trial. Pilate's wife "suffered greatly in a dream" because of Jesus's innocence, but the pharma bosses were there, so they went ahead.

It went quickly. They found a cross. However, you don't ask the King of the land (the world and more) to drag a cross! So they found a fellow named Simon, from Cyrene. Check it out, it's in Matthew, Luke, and Mark.

The Stations of the Cross ("he fell three times, received a salve from Veronica") are amazing Catholic theater. Never happened.

Was the drug industry lucrative at the time? We don't know for sure, but probably, yeah. Jesus was healing everyone for free!

"My Kingdom is not of this world". Of course not! The Kingdom is the dream, the ideal.

The big industry honchos didn't like that dream. It doesn't bring shareholder value...

But perhaps it did! The shareholder value came later, in the form of a Living Dream! The best kind!

I'm going to ask none other than Fyodr Dostoevsky to explain this shortly. (At Chapter 44, in fact.) Hang on! It's heavy.

So we surmise that the heads of corporations at that time were under Roman law. The bosses gave the orders at the trial. WAIT! It wasn't a trial then! It was a coup d'etat!

They were actually chasing Jesus since birth. The three wise Magi from Persia were Fire and Light wizards of the Legendary Beings of Light.

There is an oasis north of Cairo called the Mary (Maryam) tree. The Family stopped there for a while. There is a sycamore tree there. It's been regrafted many times but it's still there. It's a magic tree.

Mary (Magdalene) was the actual princess of the House of Bethany. She has a basilica north of Toulon. It's a fabulous place to visit.

People in the region are certain that she raised her children on that part of the coast. The Mediterranean was a large pond then, as it is today. Every major port is known to every other. The south of France had a large Hebrew community.

Her uncle Joseph was a wealthy tin merchant with a maritime fleet visiting mines in Cornwall.

Capital always talks loud. Render unto Caesar what's his. And let the King of Cooperation and Wellness be the teacher and guide He is!

Do serious healers put themselves at risk if they find basic cures for things? That's a cocktail party question if there ever was one! You must ask it!

Corporations don't like seeing their lucrative gigs get impinged upon. Imagine trying to save the world and instead of being thanked for it, you're running. No!

Urban buses have posters on them, along the top panel. Often they depict various maladies, and a foundation is fighting for a cure!

Problem is, when they find the cure, they all lose their six-figure salaries, cars, benefits, etc. Sure!

Synthetic (patented) drugs costing a penny to make and selling for 50 or 100 dollars a pop. More, you say?

Dostoevsky is screaming from off-stage right now! Go to 44 quickly if you want proof!

Lewis Carroll and Frank Baum wrote fiction, but some folks dare to suggest it was documentary!

In the Oz book, a small dog pulled the curtain away from where the wizard was controlling his fire and smoke show. Smart dog.

The jig was up. Wiz had to hand out fancy certificates, suitable for framing. Dorothy, the tin man, the scarecrow, and the lion all got their diplomas. Like a dental degree. Oh wait. Not that!

These historical accounts are vital pieces of the jigsaw puzzle towards great abundance.

Memorable people were different because they made folks laugh, but only when appropriate.

38

CHAPTER

Resurrect

Core points:

1. Saving seriously compromised teeth is always the correct approach.
2. Saving time on treatment is the wrong approach.
3. Minutes of chair-time translates to a tooth's lifetime.

Serious dental decay does not automatically have to be a root canal procedure. Many teeth can be brought back from the brink, so to speak.

There are reliable studies showing that severely necrotic teeth can also be saved. However this would require a top-quality protocol involving the use of ozone in conjunction with ART.

This area is the very pinnacle of responsive dental care and healing. If there is a tooth that's compromised right to the roots, then you've got a challenge. But even that challenge can be met successfully.

Pulp capping is necessary knowledge for all dental healers. With proficient pulp capping just about any seriously damaged tooth could be made viable. And that's the key. Viability, along with longevity.

There are terms dentists use, like pulpitis, to describe a serious dental malady that's "beyond repair". However, such severe dental injury can still be healed by using an aggressive healing protocol. Ozone has to be a key part of it.

In addition to prepping and restoring the cavity, there might be damage to the nerves of the tooth, maybe even extending to the roots.

In such a case, you're working with two things. The power of deep ozone treatment to reach into those deep tissues and do their disinfecting magic. And the ability of the body to heal itself from the inside.

These two can work together to literally bring a very injured tooth back from the precipice.

Here's a summary of the "extreme protocol" for saving very damaged teeth when 100% of dentists are calling it a root canal or an extraction:

1. The aggressive ozone therapy + ART (Atraumatic Restorative Treatment), is a pinnacle biomimetic approach.
2. For early / mild pulpitis (reversible inflammation).
3. Ozone's role: eliminates 99% of bacteria in caries, reduces inflammation via oxygenation (boosts pulp repair).
4. ART's Role: a) Seals the cavity with glass ionomer cement (GIC), which releases fluoride (antibacterial). b) Bonds to damp dentin (ideal for minimally invasive prep).
5. Outcome: Pulp can recover if blood supply is intact. 60 to 70% success in halting progression.
6. Deep caries (near-pulp exposure):
7. Ozone + partial caries removal. Avoids pulp exposure; ozone disinfects remaining infected dentin. GIC seals and stimulates tertiary dentin formation.
8. Outcome: 50% success rate in avoiding root canal (if done early).
9. Where it fails: Irreversible pulpitis or necrosis
10. Ozone's Limit: Cannot revive dead tissue or regenerate necrotic pulp. No effect on apical abscesses (root tip infection).
11. ART's Limit: GIC cannot restore pulp vitality once necrosis sets in.
12. Evidence-based alternatives for severe cases:
13. Vital Pulp Therapy (VPT) for reversible pulpitis.

14. MTA / Biodentine direct pulp capping + ozone disinfection.
15. Success rate: 75 to 90% (if pulp is vital).
16. Clinical recommendations: Best for early / moderate caries (ozone + ART), reversible pulpitis (ozone + VPT).

This is quite technical, but serious ART-based dental healers will start with this.

If you're able to do this kind of service, you will have clients lining up down the block, and maybe flying in from overseas.

You'll have ET's showing up, looking for treatment excellence. Arcturians? Maybe.

And yes, people know what a real healer looks like. It's a different animal.

So, if you're in that position and have a serious problem, a seriously injured tooth, will an ART trained dental hygienist go that far and repair it?

They're only trained in the ART protocol for superficial and shallow cavities. So it all depends.

If a hygienist uses common sense and has a sense of adventure, then yes, they will be able to save almost any tooth.

They won't be using power tools, so it's quite conceivable for them to be capable at this.

Most likely, their ART training doesn't include pulp capping. It's an extra module. So simple.

Now imagine how rewarding it is when you've brought a tooth back from the brink, and made it functional again. The sense of accomplishment would be SUPERB.

We need a stage! We need ridiculous costumes....

39

CHAPTER

Shaker 2

Hamlet Converts the Dentist: A Shakespearean dramaticule.

(Tension)

Hamlet:
"Take up a healthier means, thou confus'ed wretch!
Behold this slender wand - the ART-ist's fleche.
And tell me why thy hand still shakes for steel
Dost thou know not, the healer's weal?
O, what a rogue am I to stand and plead
When proof itself doth mock thy stubborn creed!
Minimally invasive, no white-knuckled grip,
But relief, as deft hands glide and tip.
The caries cleansed, the tooth remains unscarred,
And lo - the patient leaves thee not half-marred!"

Dentist: (*lowers drill*)
"But... speed... precision...
How can less be more?"

Hamlet:
"Less? Nay, more skill, more thought, and evermore!
The brute may swing an axe to prune a rose,
But artists touch with purpose, I suppose."

(*Dentist gazes silently. Hamlet picks up the drill.*)

Hamlet:
"This tool, inferior if truth be told.
A stressful brand, a token of the old!
Do cease to ply thy trade askance.
MID is precise, kind. O, break thy trance!"
(*Dentist staggers, as if waking from a dream. His eyes widen.*)

Dentist: (*whispering*)
"And yet I was taught...
the way of noise and pain.
T'was error for certain.
To be so proud and vain."
(*Dentist laughs. He takes the curette, weighing it in his hand.*)

Dentist:
"So light, so right. T'was but a lie -
To love the roar, and call it progress. Fie!"
(*He tosses the drill into the trash.*)

Dentist:
"Henceforth, my hand
Shall only know this dental ART,
With patients rising grateful,
Knowing that I've well played my part!"
(*Dentist beams, a man reborn*)

Hamlet: (*grinning*)
"Ay, there's the rub - thou'rt awake at last.
Now, dentist, heal. Leave the error of the past."

FIN

40

CHAPTER

Papaya

Core points:

1. Caries removal gel is pure magic.
2. The dental profession is often afraid of wonderful things.
3. The reason is that these don't directly accrue to major profits.

In the ART of dental healing, there are some magical substances. One of the very best is the gel that dissolves decay painlessly, comfortably, and effectively.

It's almost beyond magic. It's made from papaya sap. It acts on the collagen structure of caries bacteria to turn it into a very soft mush. The decayed tissue is then easily removed with a hand instrument, a dental spoon or curette.

The dental profession could be using this gel and be saving millions of people from untold pain and discomfort.

It's incomprehensible that dentists don't use this caries removal gel. They instead apply their long hypodermic needles to freeze tissue, so that they can then excavate deeply into viable tissue with their electric drills. Which causes even further damage.

Clients are terrified from start to finish. Is this dentistry? Definitely not. There's actually no name for this level of profound ignorance.

The caries removal (CR) gel removes only the decay and doesn't harm the healthy tissue in any way.

Let's dive into the detail:

1. Caries removal gel softens the infected dentin (caries) by enzyme action (papain, bromelain) or chemical agents ($NaClO$, chloramines).
2. Its chemical formula is actually really simple.
3. So simple that you could even try making some at home!
4. It selectively targets carious tissue while preserving healthy dentin.
5. It's 100% painless! (Repeat that a few times, then go straight over to your dentist and repeat it 100 times more! Gauge the reaction. Better yet, film it.)
6. Being non-invasive, it obviates mechanical drilling, and the associated pain and trauma.
7. As a painless procedure, there's no need for a terrifying needle either.
8. It's ideal for everyone but especially children (who, being kids, instinctively know that long needles are a form of legalized terror.)
9. It preserves tooth structure, healthy enamel and dentin, the opposite of drilling which often removes healthy tooth structure.)
10. It's simple to apply. Place it on caries, then after two minutes, gently scrape it away.
11. Requires only hand instruments (ART).
12. Comfort and acceptance by everyone (except by malfeasant dental boards and curriculum committees).
13. Enhances patient compliance due to no noise and vibration.
14. I could go on, but then I'd be diluting this MAGIC! Just insist on it. Stop suffering needlessly!

The biggest names on the market are Carisolv (made in Sweden) and Brix3000 (made in Argentina). There are dozens of other manufacturers, especially in China and India.

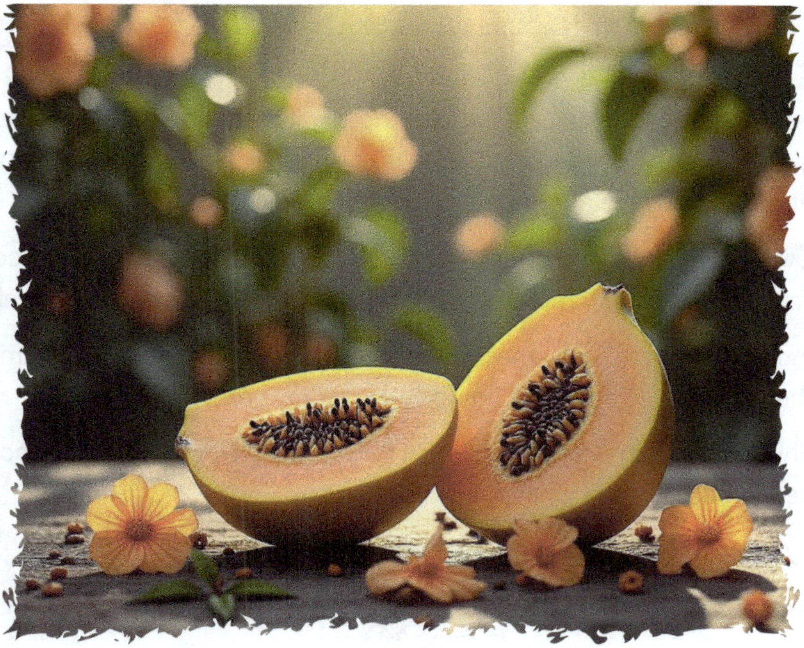

Papain is a "cysteine protease enzyme". It breaks down the decay naturally. Also:

1. It's very cheap, pennies per treatment.
2. It empowers self care, and that's no good for the business plan.
3. It's painless, and 300$ drilling jobs won't be necessary.

Dentistry is so interesting. If they found an easy cure for something, do you think they'd rush out and adopt it? Only you can answer that question for yourself. Go ahead, ask yourself. What's your answer?

Do try to obtain some CR gel for yourself as soon as you can. You'll get a great feeling of self sufficiency.

You'll be able to contemplate never having to endure a mechanical high speed drill ever again. You'll be totally elated.

Oh yes. The dentist might be fluxxomed, flabbergasted. Then, the lights will come on!

I've shown the tube of Carosolv to dentists who lecture at colleges. They never heard of it! They were keen to take a photo of it, for further investigation. Ah, the revelation.

But will they ask themselves: Why hasn't this wonder product ever been mentioned in any of the dozen trade publications they send me every week?

And why wasn't this ever mentioned at my last dental success bootcamp, where they coached me on how to max out my profit line?

Why not try to answer that question for yourself? But, you already know the reason.

In your hands is the power. Take it.

41
CHAPTER

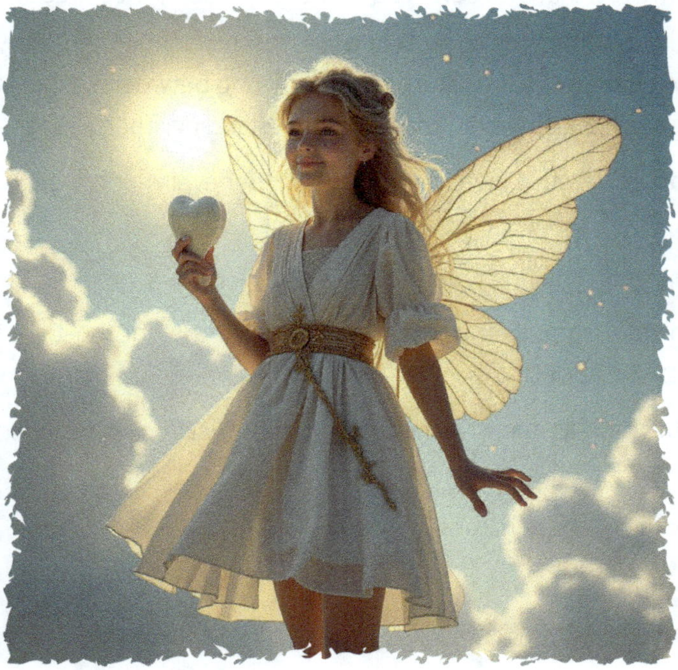

Zen Room

Core points:

1. Great oral health is not separate from wisdom.
2. Ancient people knew special things.
3. Energy is the substrate of matter.

In a traditional Zendo, you are supposed to study yourself. That's the basic idea, and it sure isn't an easy thing for many people.

If you were a dentist studying yourself (especially after returning from a week-long "dental success boot-camp"), this might indeed be a challenging process.

You'd squirm a lot, that's for sure. You'd be the one doing all the coughing.

Still, you'd have some time to relax and breathe. It's not like church, where you're listening to a lot of stuff, and alternating between sitting, standing, sitting again, maybe even kneeling, then standing. Then sitting.

In the Zendo, you just sit, period. And you ponder everything. Deep stuff.

Like:
Occlusal margins requiring tapering.

Still, you might ask yourself what light is. Not just the photon-light that science tells you about.

Some mystics have as many names for light as the Eskimos have for snow. Which is, many.

What are some of these names? We have:
Photoic
Noetic
Iatonic
Pneumatic
Uncreated

These are sometimes described as "Neoplatonic" concepts. It starts off as a knowledge state, and moves into a feeling state.

Photoic would be the light in a physical reality. Noetic would be on a knowledge level. Iatonic moves into the "true order of things". A healing order. Pneumatic is likely similar to the passions of a great artist or musician. It's a highly inspired state. Uncreated goes into areas that words do not cover.

Do they affect the dental healing path? Definitely. They are based on the premise of quantum energy. Where even material things (like teeth) have their substrate in pure energy.

latonic light is described as the healing light. It brings the situation back to its original design (or perfection). It restores.

It has been said: "Pneumatic and Uncreated Light may be the same sunlight, but now it can shine brilliantly into and through the now-clean mirror, filling the room with its radiance. The mirror not only reflects the light but seems to become light itself."

Just as a single beam of light can give birth to infinite colors (as in a prism), a Supreme Light contains the blueprint of all possibilities.

When aligned with this light, manifestation is not just about personal desires but co-creation with the universe's infinite abundance.

In this Zendo, meditation on light would clear the subconscious, allowing opportunities and wellness to arise naturally.

Science confirms that all matter is condensed light. What it doesn't say is that a certain "supreme light" is in the source code behind this phenomenon.

St. Francis spoke with birds. How he did this, few really know. But he learned the language, and it stood him well. The birds might have even advised him on optimal oral health! But we don't know for sure.

We do know that great dental wellness translates to a good feeling and a happy mindset. All the money we save (by wisely avoiding probably needless complicated dental treatments) will all go to happy and healing outcomes.

The Supreme Light doesn't just assist manifestation - it is the substance of manifestation itself.

This abundance is seen in the win-win analogy of ART. If something is a win, but it also connects to another win, then you know it's the natural way of things.

And when the land is vast, and the seasons are very sharply defined, we get some serious reflections....

42

CHAPTER

Chekhov 2

A CHEKHOVIAN SCENE

[**Setting:** A country estate at dusk. A wooden bench beneath an old oak tree in a serene garden.

Ivan Petrovich, former dentist, sits with a book by Frencken on his lap.

Maria Andreeva, his young niece, enters carrying a shawl. Golden rays of the sun filter through the leaves.]

Maria: "Are you warm enough, Uncle? The sun shall soon be gone."

Ivan: (*without looking up*) "Gone? No. It is always there. Only we turn away."

Maria: (*sitting beside him, amused*) "Spoken like an endodontist. One who now regrets."

Ivan: (*smiling faintly*) "Perhaps, Maria."

Maria: "And why, Uncle?"

Ivan: "Regret is a strong teacher, Maria."

Maria: "Please explain, Uncle."

Ivan: "I could have healed, Maria."

Maria: "You had a wonderful career!"

Ivan: "But did I heal? My brother Vasily refuses root canal procedures. He says 90% of them are unnecessary. The rest are simple extractions."

Maria: (*adjusts her shawl, sighs deeply*) "Vasily is a healer."

Ivan: "He saves teeth, Maria. I should have listened."

Maria: "But your training, Uncle…"

Ivan: "Never mentioned healing ozone, Maria. Never mentioned CR gel."

Maria: "Uncle, these are essentials. What can be done?"

Ivan: "At this stage, Maria, it's about breaking an undesirable monopoly. Allowing a healing craft to emerge. One that serves the client before serving itself."

Maria: "Uncle, shall you do this?"

Ivan: "I shall, Maria. Truth does not wait for the timid."

Maria: "You shall join your brother Vasily and design a new curriculum, Uncle?"

Ivan: "Of course, Maria."

Maria: "Then you are vibrantly renewing your purpose, Uncle!"

Ivan: "And then the regret shall flee, Maria. Perhaps forever."

Maria: "It's wonderful, Uncle."

(*The first star appears. It might be Venus! A quiet understanding hangs between them. Before them stretches the vast Russian plain.*)

CURTAIN

43

CHAPTER

The Wei

Core points:

1. Traditional Chinese Medicine has a huge missing corpus.
2. Finding the lost Wei Jing would be the greatest adventure.
3. This job posting is currently open.

When it comes to ancient knowledge, there was surely abundant wisdom regarding dental wellness. Literally vast treasures, without a doubt.

Good things do get blended, however, into the averages of time. Their husks anyway. While their spirit goes up to a higher place.

And so with dental healing. I was investigating Traditional Chinese Medicine. It's an ancient wisdom. I wanted to know how TCM approached oral health.

The Nei Jing is the oldest known text on Chinese medicine. It was compiled by the physicians and healers in the court of Huang-Di, the Yellow Emperor of China. This legendary figure is thought to be China's first king.

There is a local TCM college and I went over to see their textbooks. They have some huge ones. One is over 3000 pages thick. Almost as long as a Michener story.

To my great surprise I found only a half-page pertaining to the teeth. That was all. I knew something was very wrong here.

According to Focal Theory, the teeth account for a significant portion of the body's wellness. There should really be hundreds of pages about the health of the teeth.

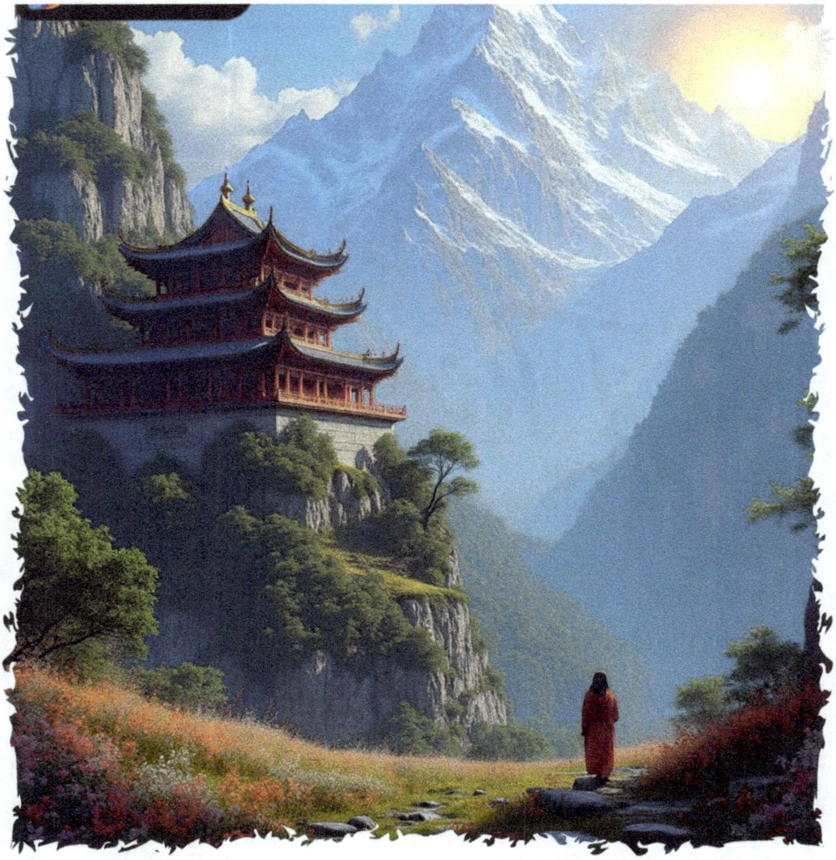

I knew I had to find the reason. Important subjects don't just get ignored. So I let it simmer on the back burner for a while.

A few days later I went over to have tea at a local shop run by a recent immigrant from China. Her name is Rainy. I asked for my small single-shot latte. She does a decent latte.

I asked her why the Nei Jing contains only a few paragraphs about the teeth.

Amazingly, she replied that the Nei Jing is only half of the corpus of TCM. Where's the other half, I asked (very excitedly).

She said: "It's missing."

"Missing?"

"Yes. It's called the Wei Jing. Nei Jing means internal medicine. The Wei Jing is all about external medicine."

I slapped that table so hard, I think I hurt myself. Whack!

"No way!"

"Yes WEI."

"But how long has it been missing?"

"Oh, maybe a few hundred years, we don't know."

I started plying Rainy with questions about where this missing text might be. Provided it still exists somewhere. We concluded that due to political turmoil, it was probably hidden in mountain caves somewhere. Or perhaps in the deep basement of some obscure monastery.

I was overjoyed to hear about this. From the local tea lady, no less.

It means that somewhere, however remote, there might be a 3000-page ancient Chinese text devoted to the healing of the teeth!

It would be an incomparable treasure!

What might this text contain? In keeping with TCM, it would be a comprehensive overview of how the body's many constituent energies play a part in keeping the teeth healthy.

TCM is mostly about energy flow. It contrasts quite vividly with western medicine.

The yin-yang, warm-cool energies all play a part. So do the body's meridians, which are like an energized circuit board for the body.

The ruling organ for the teeth are the kidneys. Strong kidney function invariably results in strong teeth.

TCM is a very intuitive medicine. Herbs are often used. These herbs are not patented profit generators. They simply work with no harmful side effects.

The Chinese often brush with special salts from a remote lake in Inner Mongolia.

What would the section on oral health in the Wei Jing look like? Can we guess?

1. It most likely has ART as its base for treatment. Hand tools, no injury.
2. Uses special clays mixed with hardeners for the restoration material.
3. Uses papatine-based formula for caries removal. This has likely been known about for millenia.
4. A greater use of herbs for pain management.
5. A long term prevention protocol using energy medicine.

In Tibetan tradition, great treasures hidden away for the benefits of future generations are called Terma Treasures. The finders of these treasures, maybe a person with a celestial calling, is called a Terton.

There is currently an open position for a person suitably qualified to go out and find the Wei Jing! Compensation will be commensurate with the magnificence of the task!

Resumes should focus on the aspirant's willingness to traverse rugged mountain ranges, sometimes on foot, enjoy barley porridge and yak butter tea, and generally have a ton of fun.

And if you do find this legendary Wei Jing, rest assured of your enduring legacy as a veritable Terton!

Meantime, we turn our attention to a modern boardroom. These executives make Jaws look like a sardine…

44

CHAPTER

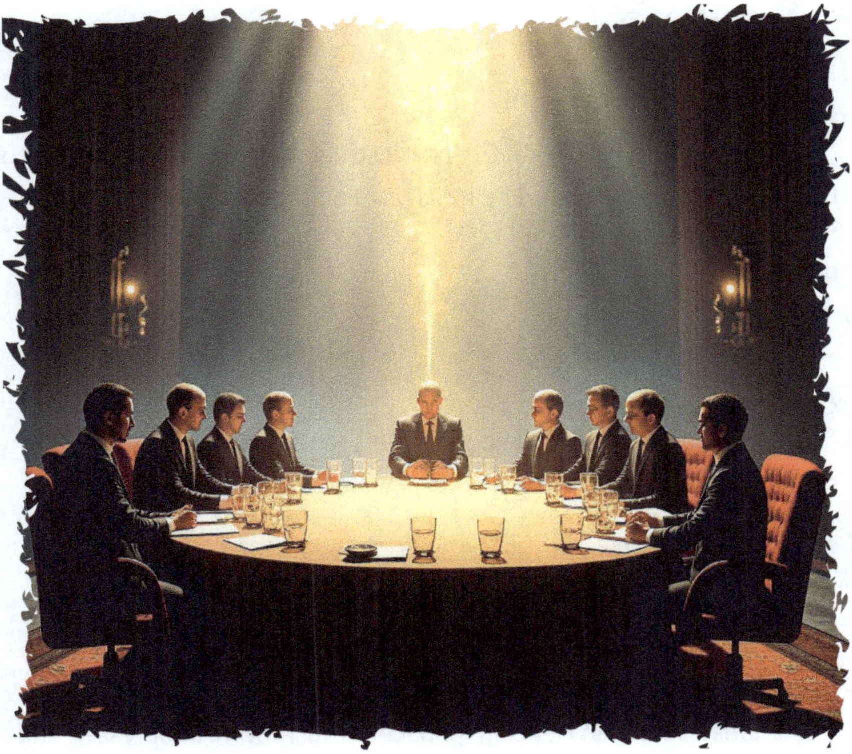

Dostoevskian

One thinks about what it might be like inside a boardroom meeting of a giant pharmaceutical company. If that thought isn't scary enough, we allow the great Dostoevsky to paint the picture:

Title: The Ledger

Zenith Pharma Boardroom. Cold light.

- Pyotr Volkov (*company CEO, 60s, gaunt, stares at the annual report to shareholders*).
- Dmitri (*CFO*),
- Anya (*Marketing*),
- Leonid (*R&D*), others.

Dmitri: (*tapping tablet*)
"Xylozap margins hit 87.4%. Co-pay restructuring worked - filtered out the... high-risk nonpayers. Life has a price point, Pyotr Alexeyevich."

Pyotr: (*eyes distant*)
"Price... yes."

Anya: (*leaning in*)
"We amplify the fear. Q4 campaign: 'Every Unchecked Cell Steals Tomorrow.' Viral dread - terrified patients pay premiums. Fear justifies cost."

Pyotr: (*fingers trembling*)
"Justifies..."

Leonid: (*sliding dossier*)
"Final update: Siberian Hericium erinaceus mushroom. Suppressed under trade laws. Was confirmed to halt early-stage Xylozap targets. Pennies per dose. We squashed it."

Pyotr: (*voice cracks*)
"Pennies...?"

Leonid:
"Patents hold. Natural cure narrative stays buried. Competitors litigate for decades. It's handled."

Pyotr:
"Handled how?"

Anya: (*impatient*)
"Pyotr Alexeyevich - focus. Fear visuals: rotting clocks? Or smiles? Which sells urgency?"

Pyotr: (*stands abruptly*)
"Sells…? You peddle terror."

Dmitri: (*cold*)
"We sell time. At fair market value."

Pyotr:
"Fair? That Siberian mushroom. It grows on trees! We did a coverup."

Leonid:
"Bioavailability required our synthetic -"

Pyotr:
"Lies! We manufactured scarcity! Patents aren't shields - they're shackles!"

Anya: (*snaps*)
"Shareholders demand growth! Fear works. If they want cheap cures, let them forage!"

Pyotr: (*sweating, gripping table*)
"All these years… a fraud. Not business - blasphemy. The mushroom spoke to me last night."

Dmitri:
"Sit down. You're unwell."

Pyotr:
"Unwell? I see the ledger! That mushroom is nature's healer."

Leonid:
"Dramatics won't -"

Pyotr:
"You think hellfire? No! It's knowing! Eternal… awareness. Floating in the void - forced to watch! Every mother bankrupted… every burial we caused… feeling their despair! Forever!"

Anya:
"Call medical. Now."

Pyotr: (*collapsing into chair*)
"The scales… they're tipping. I see it - our names. We traded lives for margins… and eternity will collect."

Dmitri: (*to speakerphone*)
"Security. Pyotr Alexeyevich is… compromised."

Pyotr: (*whispering, trembling*)
"Compromised? No. Condemned. The fraud is complete… and we'll pay… forever."

(*Pyotr stares past them, pale as bone. The dossier lies open - photos of Siberian mushrooms blooming….*)

A board meeting turned unexpectedly. Corporate shakeup on the way, with a new CEO…

45

CHAPTER

The Biohack

Core points:

1. Dental biohacking involves getting rid of false assumptions.
2. Fasting focuses the mind.
3. Healthy teeth are your birthright.

Biohacking may be a fad lately, so let's get right to the best part: the most ancient and most effective biohack must be Fasting.

Biohack is defined as: "Making strategic changes to habits and behaviors to improve things like awareness and wellness."

Fasting improves the spiritual life greatly. All the ancient religions practiced it. Many made it a core science.

The animal kingdom fasts regularly; it's how they live. Food is not always available.

Some animals can abstain from food for months at a time. Bears, when hibernating, lower their metabolism by over 90%.

Abstinence from food sharpens the mind and allows unusual lucidity. The Muslims fast during the Ramadan month (usually the hottest month of the year), not eating from sunrise to sunset.

The root word of Ramadan is thought to be "ramida" which means scorching heat. Similarly, the fast "burns away sins and purifies the believers' conscience".

The ancient Arabs fasted three days per lunar month, which they called "white days".

The early Taoists of China called their fasts Pego. They always included prayer and other exercises.

In ancient Yemen, they would fast one month per year.

The founder of Buddhism fasted intensely in order to obtain enlightenment.

Diet is a personal choice but careful thought needs to go into it. The animals raised in North American factory farming are subjected to unfathomable cruelty.

This goes directly into the convenience foods. People don't even need that food. It's mostly an unconscious habit.

Eating that material is participating in the profound cruelty cycle. In addition it sickens the body and mind.

Hippocrates, one of the founders of western medicine, recommended fasting and consuming apple cider vinegar. Ancient Greeks termed fasting "the physician within".

Conscientious biohacking is a means to wellness on many levels.

We read: "Dental biohacking moves beyond traditional dentistry to personalize treatment and may incorporate advanced diagnostics, regenerative therapies, and ozone to enhance healing and preventive care."

The hobbits are probably the ultimate biohackers, even if they don't know what the word means! They grow their own food and they don't rush around too much.

They know that a good pot of tea solves a million things.

Teeth should not be so difficult to repair and keep well. It's all in the perception.

Dentistry warns you with great alarm that you shouldn't be trying self-treatment. They might yell about "sterilization and infection control".

For hobbits, self treatment is entirely logical when done correctly and soberly. It's also 100% legal. The legal grey area is when they are treated by a non-licensed friend or family member.

Meantime, in Tijuana, a cynical comic found revelation and his world got jolted in a nice way....

46

CHAPTER

Prioritizing

George Carlin, wry cynical comedian who was afraid of dentists for 20 years, finds Richard Pryor, who has reinvented himself as an ART atraumatic dentist.

Pryor's clinic is at Plaza Zapato in the Zona Rio of Tijuana. George relaxes on the sofa after a relaxing treatment.

Richard Pryor = RP
George Carlin = GC

RP: Them mf's wouldn't let me in that dental college. So I had to go to Tanzania and learn it there. Instead of four years it was two months. Tuition? Less than one percent including airfare and room and board at the Safari.

GC: And you think you can do dentistry better now?

RP: Beats all them suckers who paid for four years of shit.

GC: Well, your atraumatic restorative treatment did a damn good job on my chompers last week. That's why I came back.

RP: And they told you you'd need six root canals and crowns, right?

GC: I was quoted five grand on it.

RP: And I charged you three hundred.

GC: That's right, Richie. That's right. I gotta be careful I don't call you boy.

RP: Boy don't matter. It's better than some of the other street shit I'm hearing.

GC: Wayyyyy better.

RP: Listen George. You got in deep, deep shit for going too close to the dark empire. And they don't like that. Let me tell you, I'm not black. I'm soul. My color is pure light.

GC: I knew that, Richard. I knew it.

RP: Yah. When they try and pull that color shit on everyone, they just do that to divide and conquer. That's why I'm pure light, George. I identify as sunshine, buddy.

GC: You are damn sunshine, boy! Oops. I mean, you work good and cheap, Richard. You just did four high quality restorations and you didn't even have to drill.

RP: That's my ART, George.

GC: That's your ART, Richard. Besides, your hyper-vulgar swearing is better with a gentle scrape than with a shrieking whine after a long needle.

RP: You got that right, George. And your deep hippie brooding goes better with a genuine smile than with a synthetic full mouth reconstruction smile at 30 grand.

GC: Richard, how long you gonna keep this gig going? You're not even licensed by the boards.

RP: I'm licensed by the stand up comedy board, and that's the only board that matters.

GC: You're totally right, Richard. Totally right.

RP: Cash or card, George?

47

CHAPTER

Peroxide

Core points:

1. Hydrogen Peroxide is a proven disinfectant.
2. It assists periodontal wellness.
3. All dental clinics can be engaged with on levels of healthiness.

Summary: Hydrogen peroxide, diluted to a 4% solution, makes an effective and cleansing mouthwash with disinfecting properties and no side effects.

I've been using hydrogen peroxide for quite a while now. It's really amazing stuff. Use food-grade only.

You purchase it concentrated at about a 50% solution, which is actually quite harmful. It'll burn everything.

You need to dilute it down to about 3 or 4% using good clean spring water, the best quality water possible.

It's really effective. It tastes a bit like bleach, which shouldn't put you off because it's pure oxygenated water.

No other elements except pure hydrogen and oxygen. The oxygen has the extra ozone molecule, so we write it as H_2O_2.

Oxygen is the greatest healer. Athletes use hyperbaric chambers with concentrated oxygen to heal quickly so they can get back on the playing field as quickly as possible. They're being paid millions to help their team!

It actually has many uses for disinfecting. You can soak vegetables or fruit in a hydrogen peroxide bath and it works. No chemicals!

For good oral hygiene:

1. Whitens Teeth. Gently removes surface stains by oxidizing discolored molecules, making teeth appear brighter.
2. Eliminates harmful bacteria. Acts as an antimicrobial agent, reducing bacteria that cause plaque, gingivitis, and bad breath.
3. Treats gum problems. Reduces gum issues as it eliminates bacteria in periodontal pockets.
4. Freshens breath. Neutralizes odor-causing bacteria, providing a deep clean beyond regular brushing.
5. Reduces plaque buildup. When used as a mouthwash, it helps break down biofilm (plaque) on teeth and gums.
6. Disinfects toothbrushes. Soak your toothbrush. You will see a lot of fizzing and bubbles. It's a high efficiency cleaning of all the bacteria!

Swish some hydrogen peroxide after brushing to really remove all the gummy biofilm! It will quickly become part of your essential oral wellness toolkit!

Now we step out again, to visit a dental office and ask where they rate on a scale from one to ten, for healthiness. (One is an upselling crown mill, and ten is the very healthiest.)

The receptionist will often say:

"We're a 10. Of course!".

Then ask: "Do you use ozone here?"

"Uh, what's that?"

"It's 99.9% effective for eliminating harmful bacteria, with zero side-effects, when used correctly. Heals and regenerates tissue. Essential for anyone who's had an RCT."

"Oh, really?"

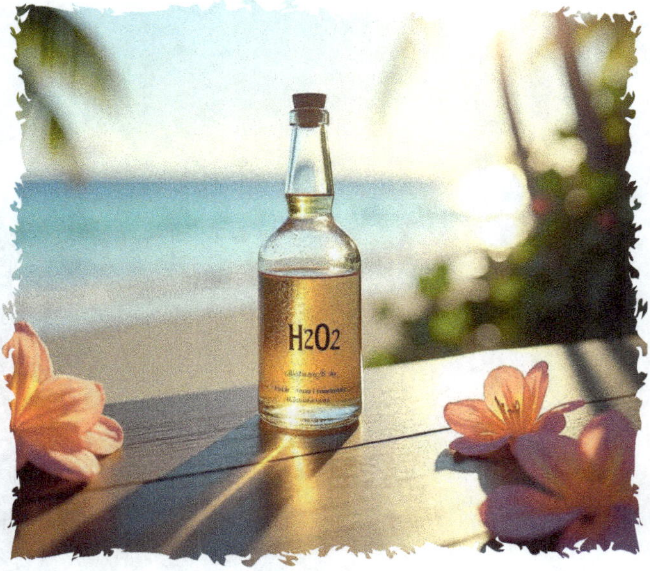

"Sorry, you're a 9 now."

"Ouch."

"Do you have CR gel here?"

"Uh, what's that?"

"Safe, effective, painless removal of dental caries. No harmful side effects. No sedation required."

"Oh... Really!"

"Are you an 8 now?"

"Oh, darn."

"Did I mention hydrogen peroxide yet?"

"Not yet."

"Hmmm. 7. Should I stop now?"

"No. Please. Keep going!"

Certain explorers of the abstracted realms could be forgiven for being passionate about dental healing theory...

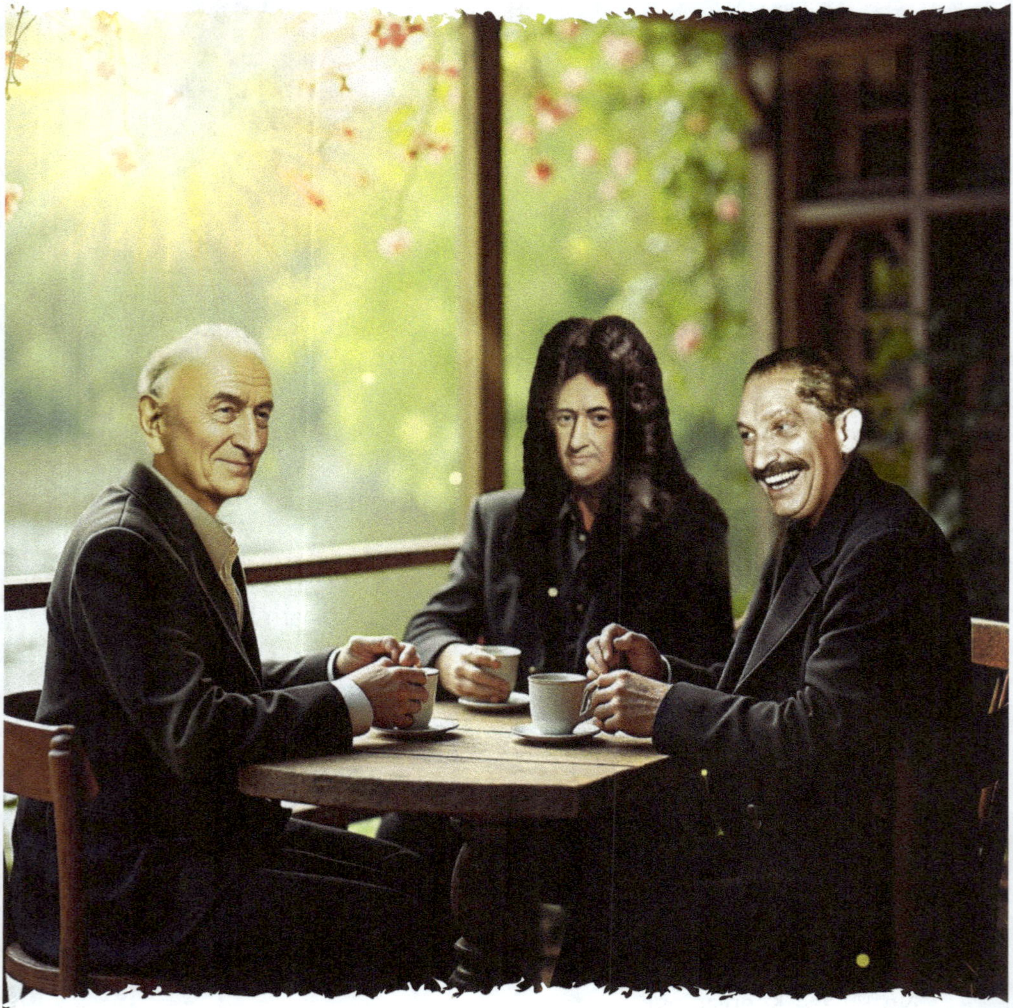

48

CHAPTER

Ein Kaffeehaus 3

Three dentist-philosophers meet at a terrace cafe in Erfurt. Gottfried Leibniz, Martin Heidegger, and Karl Jaspers. They take a small worn, wooden table next to the Gera river. Hot drinks arrive.

Leibniz: (*stirring his cappuccino with precise, energetic motions*) "This lovely reflected light on the Gera has me thinking of ideal oral health."

Heidegger: "Doof. You're a secret dentist. As we all are!"

Leibniz: "A sublime calculus."

Jaspers: "Not exactly. More like a tenuous limit-situation with a risk of dangerous exposure."

Heidegger: "What danger?"

Jaspers: "I refuse to do root canal treatments. I prefer to save every tooth. Now I might lose academic tenure."

Leibniz: "Definitely NOT the best of all possible worlds!"

Heidegger: "Herr Karl, there are many options available for saving teeth. But the "standards of care" (*based on the dummkopf curriculum*) ignores these!"

Jaspers: "And it's we, the dentists, who are blamed!"

Leibniz: "This calculus is troubling. Perhaps dentists need to know better that their training is very corporate in nature, and avoids the many creative healing opportunities."

Heidegger: "Yet this stark fact might crush their entire business structure."

Jaspers: "Not necessarily, Herr Martin. Business always finds a way to adapt to realistic circumstances."

Leibniz: (*stands abruptly*) "But these circumstances are the very notions of optimal health and wellness!"

Heidegger: "Truly so, Gotty. It's the unconcealment - aletheia."

Leibniz: "It's much more!" (*paces, very agitated*) "It's nothing less than the truth itself."

Jaspers: "Frau Muller consulted ten dentists and all of them recommended an RCT. She then came to me and had a comfortable ART restoration with a biomimetic pulp-cap. Wonderfully simple! Now her distal molar shall live a very long time!"

Leibniz: "Genius, Herr Karl. Simply genius."

Heidegger: "Normal standard of care for a dental healer! The Dasein of fully engaged participation."

Leibniz: "And yet, labeled pseudo-science to the dental boards and curriculum designers!"

Heidegger: "And this is why we consume alcoholic beverages!"

Leibniz: "In copious amounts. Because of the Christmas music also."

Heidegger: "Oh, those same 20 songs over and over?"

Leibniz: "Drunken crooners!"

Jaspers: "Lichtung! We must clear away the false."

Leibniz: "PROST!"

(*A silence falls, filled with birdsong. The mist thins over the slow moving river.*)

49

CHAPTER

Excellence

Core points:

1. A dental anthropologist discovered excellent oral health.
2. Pure-state unprocessed foods were the key.

"Here's my passport, Sir."

"Purpose of your visit?"

"Your people like taro and coconut. I need to interview them."

"Here's your stamp. Please stay out of trouble."

Imagine taking two years to travel all around the world, searching for people with perfect teeth! Someone actually did this a century ago. He was a dental anthropologist named Weston Price.

This fellow was the Indiana Jones of teeth! He brought journals with him, and filled them with jokes, and also with notes.

Price travelled during the 1930's. His findings included:

1. Isolated groups eating traditional diets had almost no cavities. Those eating processed foods (sugar, white flour) rapidly developed decay.
2. Healthy traditional diets (rich in fat-soluble vitamins) led to broad dental arches, straight teeth, and wide faces with enough room for wisdom teeth.
3. Importance of fat-soluble vitamins (A, D, K2). Found in butter and fermented foods. Crucial for strong bones, teeth, and immune health.
4. Soil health = human health: Mineral-rich soils produce nutrient-dense foods, leading to healthier teeth and bodies in traditional societies.

5. Raw and fermented foods were key: Indigenous diets included raw dairy, and soaked grains.
6. Dental health reflects overall health.
7. Modern food processing destroyed nutrition: Refined sugars, vegetable oils, and pasteurized foods compromised wellness.
8. Preventive nutrition over dentistry: Price argued that proper nutrition could prevent dental problems better than fillings or braces.

This is powerful stuff. The raw vegan diet seems to be strongly vindicated by this.

Processed, manufactured food is not the same living food as raw natural food is. It's missing much of that vitality. And yet, do many people care? A bit maybe.

Ulla Schmid has a website called "Healing Teeth Naturally". She says:

1. "Remineralizing means forming new hardened enamel.
2. Such remineralization or "glazing over" of teeth is best achieved by a nutrition rich in minerals, trace elements, vitamins and various phytonutrients.
3. Avoid refined and other damaging foodstuffs, especially sugar and white flour."

Snack foods carry a price, named Weston! To be a food purist, you might have to forgo the easy fun for a while. It's going to be damn tough. So much advertising goes into it.

Or maybe you want to go full Paleo and return to your primitive roots in a forest or jungle. Building a shelter from sticks and forest debris.

But first, let Weston show by his experience that excellent teeth are possible. Even if you don't have a time machine.

50

CHAPTER

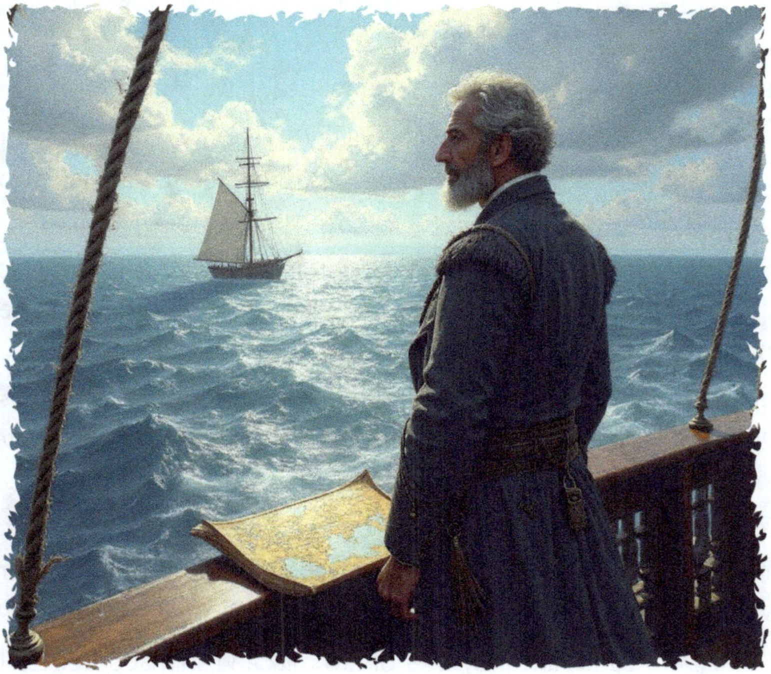

Adventure

Core points:

1. Some isolated communities thrived without professional dentistry.
2. No one "worked over" their teeth with mechanical tools.

Weston Price traveled with a serious purpose. Many years ago, I traveled mostly for fun and adventure. These days, I tend to travel mostly for fun and adventure.

Traveling the way Weston Price did, in search of people with perfect teeth, is something that very few people would actually think of doing. Until they find out that it's a very smart travel plan. Then the passion begins.

So where exactly did Weston Price find people with great teeth? Definitely not in convenience stores full of soda pop and other unmentionables.

Price made discoveries of excellent dental health with:

1. Swiss alpine villagers (Loetschental Valley): Diet of raw milk, cheese, rye bread, some meats. Virtually no cavities, broad dental arches, strong immunity.
2. Gaelic fishermen (Outer Hebrides, Scotland): Diet of oats, fish (especially cod liver), shellfish, limited dairy. No tooth decay, and no need for dentists, strong bones.
3. Native Americans and Inuit (Northern Canada, Florida Everglades): Diet of wild game, fish, corn (nixtamalized), squash, beans. Perfect teeth in pre-modern groups; decay followed contact with settlers.
4. Polynesians (South Pacific islands): Diet of seafood, coconut, taro, fermented breadfruit. No cavities in traditional groups; decay appeared with trade foods.
5. Masai (Kenya and Tanzania): Diet of raw milk and animal products. No decay and no dentists.
6. Australian aborigines: Diet of kangaroo, seafood, insects, wild plants. No decay in hunter-gatherers; dental problems with processed diet.
7. New Zealand Māori: Diet of shellfish, fern roots. (pre-European contact). Strong teeth and jaws before processed foods.
8. Peruvian indigenous (Andes Mountains): Diet of quinoa, potatoes, alpaca meat, fish (dried). No cavities in remote villages; decay in cities.
9. Melanesians (Solomon Islands, Fiji): Diet of seafood, coconut, yams. Perfect teeth where diets were traditional.

These are serious findings. You want to buy a ticket and go there. However, these are places in the past. Or could they be part of the present?

Weston Price's research inspired the ancestral health and Paleo movements. These movements are mostly peaceful, but become militant, perhaps even violent, when denied their basic wants.

Price paid the price, and now he is often quoted. Those quotes generate ad revenue. But the bottom line is that he knew that snack foods carry a silent watcher. This watcher ought to leave the room immediately. A showdown is brewing.

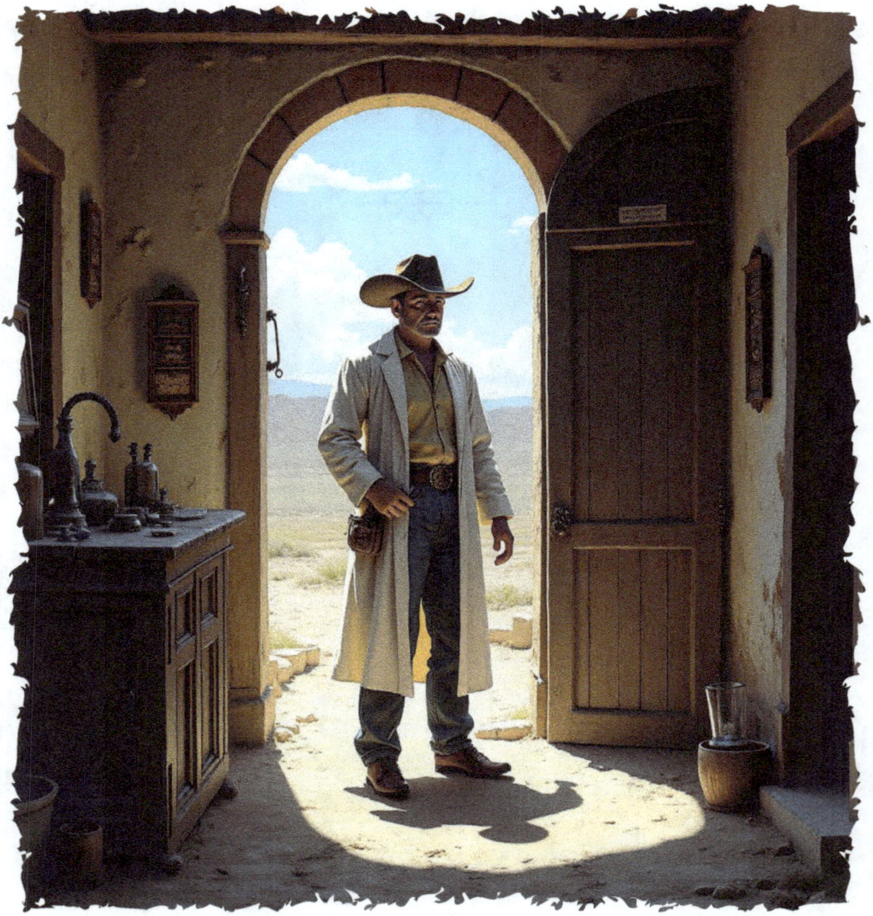

51

CHAPTER

Showdown!

Title: "The Gel of San Miguel"

Setting:

A baking hot frontier town. The Dentistería del Oro clinic sits at the end of the only street, its swinging sign creaking in the wind. Inside, the air is thick with the scent of whiskey and iron.

Three invasive dentists (Stony, Snakey, and Knuckles) brutish men in dirty aprons, work like cheap mechanics, their tools crude, their methods merciless. Patients scream. Teeth are wrenched with pliers. Gold fillings are piled like loot on a table.

On the edge of town, a lone figure appears.

Dr. Charles Bronson, roaming ART atraumatic dentist, walks deliberately up the dusty road to the clinic, pauses, then steps inside. Closeup on boots. Walks to a corner and settles himself. His instruments gleam. His hands move like a card sharp's. He doesn't speak.

Picks up harmonica. Begins to play a long single note. The long note rises and falls without break; it's haunting. After a minute, very slowly puts down the harmonica. Looks up to the others.

"You Frank?"

(*a one minute pause*)

"We're Frank's endodontists."

"Got room in your clinic for ART?"

"ART…?" (*they all laugh uproariously*)

Now, a terrified rancher is dragged in, his jaw covered. They reach for their biggest pliers.

Snakey (*grinning*):

"This one's gonna sing!"

Dr. Bronson watches. Then -

A single, deliberate click as he sets down a sterilized explorer. The sound cuts through the room like a gunshot. The laughter stops.

Story (*sneering*):

"You gonna do somethin', fancy hands?"

Dr. Bronson stands. Slow, unhurried. He approaches the rancher, eyes locked on the aching molar. The other dentists raise their tools like weapons as they step back.

Closeup on Dr. Bronson's hands, as he administers a cocaine solution, just enough. A single background guitar note for each movement. He quickly scrapes with a curette, and places a clean composite restoration before the others have time to react.

"Never seen pulp cap before?"

The rancher gets up quickly, looks around, then bolts.

Now the endodontists move in slowly, like a jackal pack.

Snakey (*muttering*): "Ain't natural."

Dr. Bronson starts cleaning his instruments as the other dentists flinch. They've seen ART, it terrifies them. The town's windmill groans. They raise their drills.

Dr Bronson steps back and shakes his head slowly from side to side (*an unmistakable* "No"...)

A new patient, a young vaquero walks in.

Snakey: "Eh, artista? You gonna watch, or you gonna do that nothin' you do?"

Dr. Bronson deliberately unscrews a vial of Filtek composite.

Stony (*squinting*): "Da heck is that?"

Dr. Bronson leans in to work.

After a minute, the vaquero asks: "I no feel. When you start?"

Dr. Bronson: (*slowly*) "Done."

"Ehhhhh…?" The man bolts up. Reaches in his pocket and offers a large gold escudo. Dr. Bronson pauses, then reluctantly accepts it.

Dr. Bronson: "Could use an aperitif, an avocado roll with miso, and a bed for the night. Do they carry Investors Weekly here?"

Snakey reacts. "We got a special bed for strangers like you." Cocks his drill and moves in quickly.

Dr. Bronson is faster. A boot to the crotch drops Snakey like a sack of spuds.

The others draw back.

Dr. Bronson picks up the harmonica. Another long single note…

Commotion outside. A crowd has assembled, rushing up and eager to get treated.

Stony and Knuckles spit hard. They run up to snatch the gold fillings on the table. They leave out the back door, dragging Snakey with them.

A janitor steps up. "Looks like you mighta won yerself a clinic."

Dr. Bronson slowly puts down the harmonica. "Where do I find Frank?"

A tumbleweed rolls past the group outside.

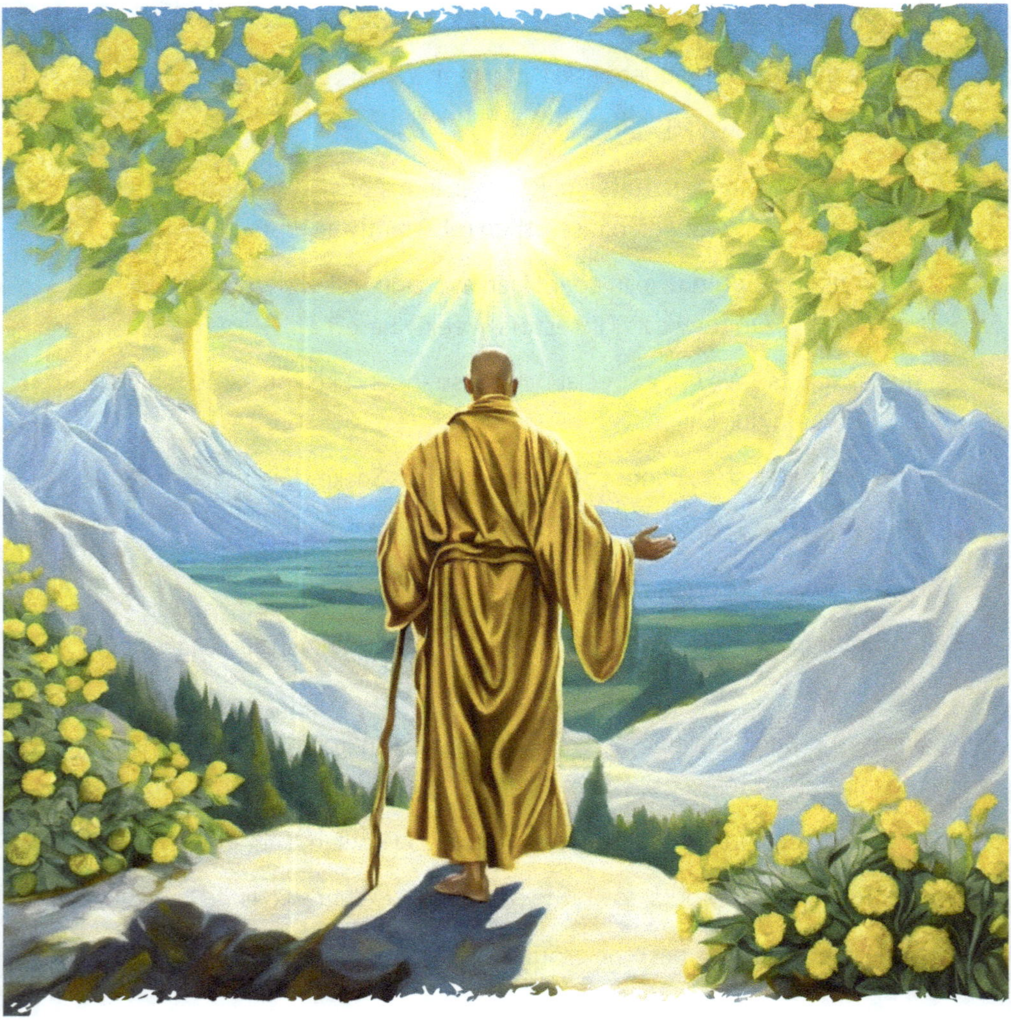

A new patient, a young vaquero walks in.

Snakey: "Eh, artista? You gonna watch, or you gonna do that nothin' you do?"

Dr. Bronson deliberately unscrews a vial of Filtek composite.

Stony (*squinting*): "Da heck is that?"

Dr. Bronson leans in to work.

After a minute, the vaquero asks: "I no feel. When you start?"

Dr. Bronson: (*slowly*) "Done."

"Ehhhhh…?" The man bolts up. Reaches in his pocket and offers a large gold escudo. Dr. Bronson pauses, then reluctantly accepts it.

Dr. Bronson: "Could use an aperitif, an avocado roll with miso, and a bed for the night. Do they carry Investors Weekly here?"

Snakey reacts. "We got a special bed for strangers like you." Cocks his drill and moves in quickly.

Dr. Bronson is faster. A boot to the crotch drops Snakey like a sack of spuds.

The others draw back.

Dr. Bronson picks up the harmonica. Another long single note…

Commotion outside. A crowd has assembled, rushing up and eager to get treated.

Stony and Knuckles spit hard. They run up to snatch the gold fillings on the table. They leave out the back door, dragging Snakey with them.

A janitor steps up. "Looks like you mighta won yerself a clinic."

Dr. Bronson slowly puts down the harmonica. "Where do I find Frank?"

A tumbleweed rolls past the group outside.

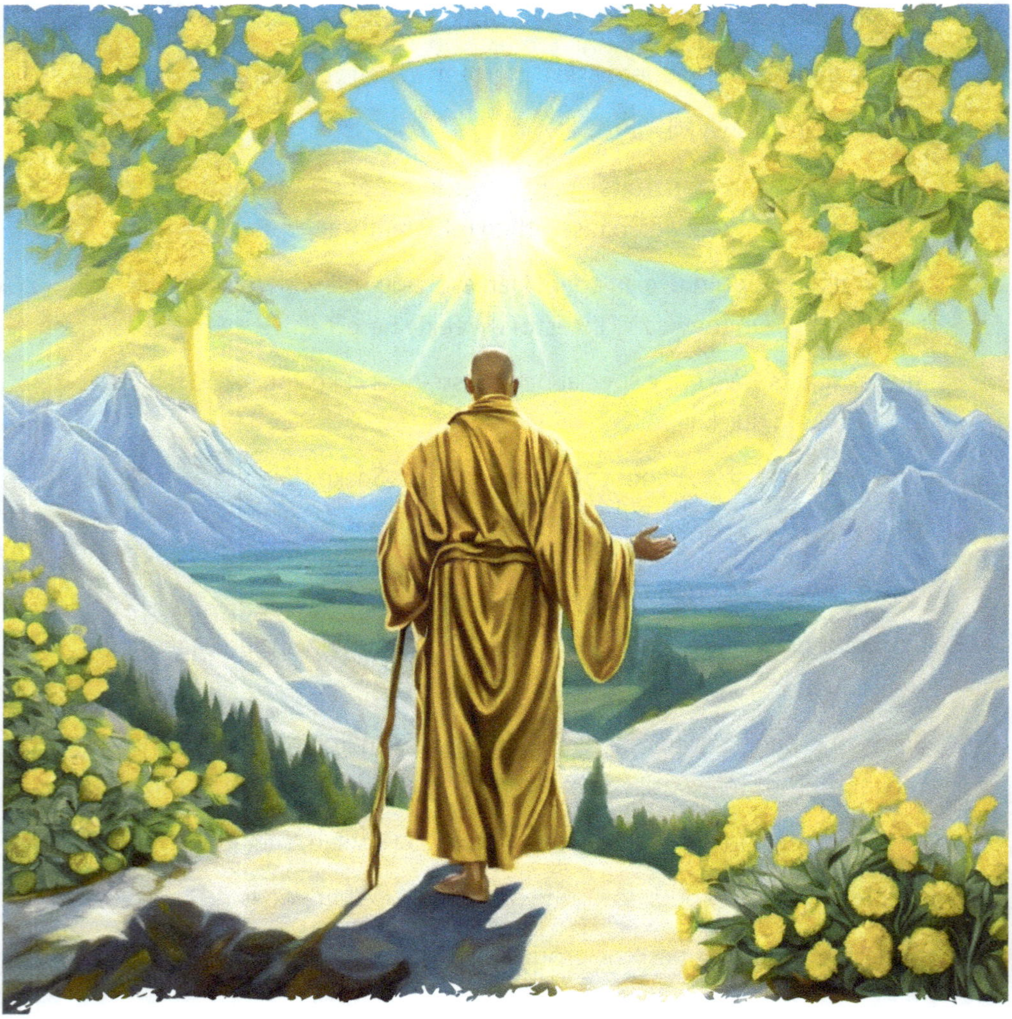

52

CHAPTER

B2 Study

Core points:

1. Brännström was a pioneer in studying the risks of dental drills.
2. Drill-free dentistry is strongly validated.
3. Dentists benefit by providing a healing practice.

We have more studies proving the definite harm done to living teeth by mechanical drilling! Dental longevity goes in the opposite direction!

A 1965 paper by Dr. Martin Brännström of Sweden was a groundbreaker:

1. Heat generation: High-speed drills (even with water cooling) cause thermal injury to the pulp, risking necrosis.
2. Microcracks in dentin: Aggressive drilling creates micro-fractures, weakening tooth structure long-term.
3. Smear layer problems: Drill friction produces a smear layer that blocks dentinal tubules, impairing adhesion and increasing sensitivity.
4. Pulp inflammation: Even "safe" drilling distances can trigger reversible pulpitis due to vibration and heat.
5. Dentin permeability changes: Drilling opens dentinal tubules, increasing fluid movement and post-op sensitivity.
6. Cavity margin damage: Over-preparation leads to enamel cracks, increasing microleakage risk.
7. Traumatic occlusion: Over-drilled teeth are more prone to cracks under biting forces.

8. Less is more: Preserving affected dentin (slightly demineralized but sterile) is better than over-cutting.
9. Hand instruments are safest: Manual excavation causes minimal pulp irritation compared to burs.
10. Vibration trauma: High-speed drills transmit harmful mechanical vibrations to the pulp.
11. Secondary caries risk: Poorly sealed drill margins lead to recurrent decay.
12. Adhesive dentistry limits: Smear layer from drilling reduces bond strength of composites.
13. Alternative methods are needed: Brännström advocated for air abrasion, enzymes, and chemo-mechanical caries removal (later developed as Carisolv).
14. Prevention over restoration: Emphasized early caries interception to avoid caries.

Brännström shook the foundations of corporate dentistry. But like an earthquake at Richter 2, they collectively went "Huh?..." and then mostly carried on as before.

Some listened, though. New studies soon came out that focused on lessening the existing drill damage.

These seem to have been sponsored by the drill manufacturers as a way to lessen the obvious harms of their products. Makes sense.

What these studies really did was to confirm the vastly superior benefits of the ART protocol!

This evidence needs to be presented to packed seminars in upper level dental college!

(Warning: Do not attempt this if the faculty hasn't been briefed about it! And do not attempt it while wearing only briefs either!)

If the dentist knows about these studies, will he continue to use the drill? A good way to find out is to present them to your own dentist.

We have some provocative sample dentist letters at Chapters 61 and 67. Dare the reality show!

Dentists by and large mean well within the framework of their training. They clearly think they're helping people and doing them a service. They simply don't know.

They are trained in a way that causes progressive tooth injury. That's the stark fact.

Their curriculum, the one they spent tens of thousands of dollars to learn over four years, taught them an invasive dentistry that doesn't seriously comprehend tooth longevity.

Dentists need to have the toolkit for true healthy and trauma-free dentistry. And that toolkit is called ART.

A clear win-win situation for both the dentist and the client. At least when coherence prevails.

In certain instances, however, coherence gives way to a sort of uncharted verbal landscape....

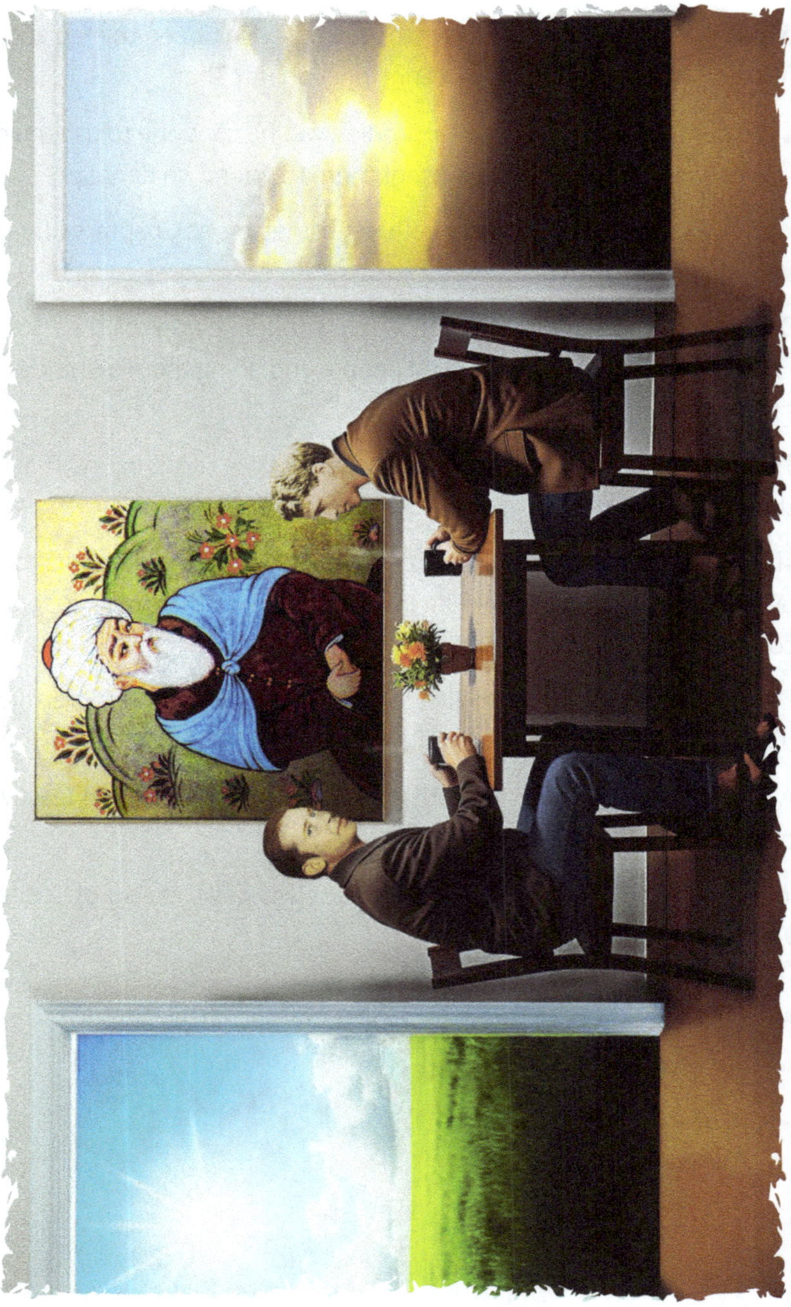

53 CHAPTER

RF & ee

Core points:

1. Dental fluoride has a dual nature.
2. It's very toxic if ingested.
3. It might enable the formation of "fluoro-apatite", a decay-resistant re-mineralization.

A breeze is blowing the scattered clouds across a sunlit sky. Poet-dentist Robert Frost (RF) meets renegade healer ee cummings (ee) at the Caffe Rumi, across the road from the Fairview Dental Center in a large urban location.

Frost sips a latte while cummings has a croissant and an orange juice.

RF: (takes a sip) You have been one, acquainted with the ART.
You are now done with pain,
Have returned in gain.
You have out-walked the furthest dental cart.

ee: (dental)
(contractsmiles)
ad(justing)
yes.
one
ac(quainted) with the
(f.r.i.g.h.t.)

a
c
c
o
o
u
n
t
s
(rec'vbles)
ledgered in
chair
time

RF: You have looked on the saddest occlusal bitewing.
Been examined by the endodontic assistant
Dropped your eyes, unwilling to proceed.

ee: o
but
the
(real)
work-
the painless
the
effective
the
true
a. trau
matic

RF: You have stood still, stopped the sound of error,
In the next operatory, an interrupted cry
From a drill, wrongly applied.

ee: (o the
slick
brochure
promises)
(while the
lidocain
wears
off
before
the
payment
plan)

RF: And not to console, or to heal you back.
And further still, the bill, an unearthly sum.
Folded before ART's correctness.

ee: (the
client
t
o
o
oft
a
profit
center
com(pliant)
in
the
(chair)
dis-earn
a.
b

e
t
t
e
r
(way)

RF: Proclaimed: you shifted, from wrong to right.
You truly have been one, acquainted with the ART.

ee: it's
a
s.t.a.r.t.)

[**note 1**: ee paid the bill for this encounter with
m
o
n
e
y
.]

[**note 2**: a beauty of this exchange is that it makes all other typographical errors in this entire volume completely acceptable as "pieces of art".]

[**note 3**: the fourth wall must never be broken.]

54

CHAPTER

Fluorides

There is a compelling debate regarding the use of fluoride in dentistry.

It seems to distill into two basic points:

1. When ingested, fluoride is a powerful poison.
2. Fluoride can beneficially bond with the calcium and phosphate ions in the tooth's enamel to form a very strong "fluoro-apatite". This is more resistant to decay than normal dental enamel.

The debate seems to be best resolved when ingestion is avoided completely, and when topical (external) use of fluoride is carefully and wisely used.

Bacteria in the mouth are seen as plaque. They consume sugars and produce acids. This acid dissolves the main mineral of the enamel, which is a crystal called hydroxy-apatite. The chemical formula for this enamel is: $Ca_{10}(PO_4)_6(OH)_2$.

Saliva is slightly basic (alkaline) and contains calcium (Ca) and phosphate (PO_4) ions.

In between acidic attacks, it washes these minerals back over the tooth, trying to rebuild the dissolved crystals. It's a constant tug-of-war.

Fluoride might positively incorporate itself into the crystal structure, replacing the hydroxide (OH^-) ion to form a new, much stronger mineral called fluoro-apatite ($Ca_{10}(PO_4)_6F_2$).

Key points:

1. Hydroxy-apatite dissolves in a mild acid (pH 5.5).
2. Fluoro-apatite requires a much stronger acid (pH 4.5) to dissolve.
3. It indicates that the fluoride-treated tooth can withstand a more acidic environment before it starts to decay.

This is the argument for topical use of fluoride. The argument against fluoride is directed at its high toxicity when actually ingested.

A well respected doctor named Lawrence Wilson says:

1. Fluorides are all highly toxic for the body.
2. Water fluoridation is a total abomination.
3. Problems with artificial fluoridation at "safe levels" include allergic reactions, fluorosis (fluoride poisoning), and many more.
4. Fluoride is a by-product of the aluminum and fertilizer industries.

Wilson is pointing directly to water fluoridation, which results in needless ingestion of toxic fluoride. He is less convincing regarding topical (non ingested) use.

An investigation in Australia said:

1. Fluoride is a basic ingredient of nerve gas.
2. Sodium fluoride is a hazardous waste byproduct from the manufacture of aluminum and phosphate fertilizer.
3. It's a common ingredient in rat and cockroach poisons, anesthetics, hypnotics, psychiatric drugs, and military nerve gas.
4. It has always been quite expensive to properly dispose of.
5. Some aluminum industries with an overabundance of it sold it to be put into public water supplies.
6. Since people only drink 0.5% of the total water supply, the rest simply goes down the drain as free hazardous-waste disposal for the chemical industry.

This study indicates that these chemical industries pounced upon a money-saving opportunity. It smells of deception.

Other reputable studies on fluoride toxicity include:

1. Martinetz (1980s): In "Fluoride: The Freedom Fight", toxicologist David Martinetz reiterated that fluoride "inhibits enzymes, damages cells, and disrupts energy production."
2. Christopher Bryson, in the book "The Fluoride Deception" is clearly calling the issue a large-scale fraud.

The premise behind water fluoridation is ridiculous in the first place. When water is drunk, it hardly even touches the teeth. Is it supposed to pass through the digestive tract and somehow make it back up to the teeth? Doh...

The whole idea hasn't been thought out at all, yet there they are poisoning water with it.

Topical (non-ingested) fluoride is obviously the only way to go. Its potential for enamel strengthening is compelling.

For this, you'd have a choice of fluoridated toothpaste, or using a dental tray. The latter makes much more sense, as it's controlled and specific.

[Disclaimer: This is informational only, not advice. Consult a professional always.]

A dental tray would hold a special gel of stannous fluoride, which is an enhanced compound with tin. (Tin is "stannum" in Latin.)

The objective would be to saturate the surface of the teeth with the fluoride gel for a short period, around 10 minutes. Then, the denatured enamel would form a bond to result in fluoro-apatite, which is reinforced enamel.

Always consult with a professional healer on this and obtain multiple opinions.

The fluoride amount used in GIC composite (used in ART) is deemed small enough to pose no realistic danger.

By understanding the actual effects of fluoride, we can decide exactly where it belongs in dentistry. Fluoride use is at an interesting crossroads.

It promises to strengthen dental enamel, but at the same time carries definite toxicity risk if ingested.

Now that we're talking toothpaste, are we ready for the very best?

55

CHAPTER

Dentifrice

Core points:

1. Making your own toothpaste is easy and enjoyable.
2. You choose exactly what goes into it.
3. Many commercial toothpastes contain harmful ingredients.

People with awesome dental health take really good care of their teeth. It's a skill they have! And they don't skimp on oral hygiene.

When they buy toothpaste (dentifrice) they get the best!

However, what if you could leapfrog these jet-setters and supermodels, and have an even better dentifrice? No way!

Hold on. The super brilliant way is simply to make your own! This way you have a custom designed product that's exactly what you're looking for.

The two foundations of your custom designed dentifrice are: coconut oil and baking soda. Both magic!

Nadine Artemis describes what's in many of the big brand dentifrices:

1. Fluoride, of course, which is very controversial. It might be rat poison! Study it.
2. An auto antifreeze called propylene glycol. Nice!
3. FD&C colour pigments.
4. Agent orange, also known as triclosan. Smells like war!

5. Artificial sweeteners. Oh, great. We need everything to be sweet!
6. Ethanol, a petroleum solvent. Fun!
7. Detergents and foaming agents. Of course!
8. Trisodium phosphate, an industrial degreaser. Need to get that grease out!
9. Carbomer, a gasoline polymer used to thicken. Rev that engine!
10. Hydrated silica, an abrasive. Dang. Everything on this list is abrasive or toxic! Who ever knew!

Instead of these, Artemis recommends:

1. Sea buckthorn berry.
2. Tea tree.
3. Cinnamon.
4. Neem.
5. Oregano.

These are very different. Wonderful healing herbs. They're options for adding to your two foundation substances:

1. Organic coconut oil.
2. Baking soda.

Take one cup each and mix them together well. You might need to soften or liquefy the coconut oil by placing it in a pot of hot water. When you're done mixing, then add your essential oils.

I personally prefer tea tree oil. It's super curative and disinfectant. Use around 10 drops. It's very strong.

For flavoring, try essential peppermint, clove, or oregano. Concentrated oregano has long been used by dental healers to ward off cavities.

Stir your product well. Once you have your first batch of homemade dentifrice, you will be elated.

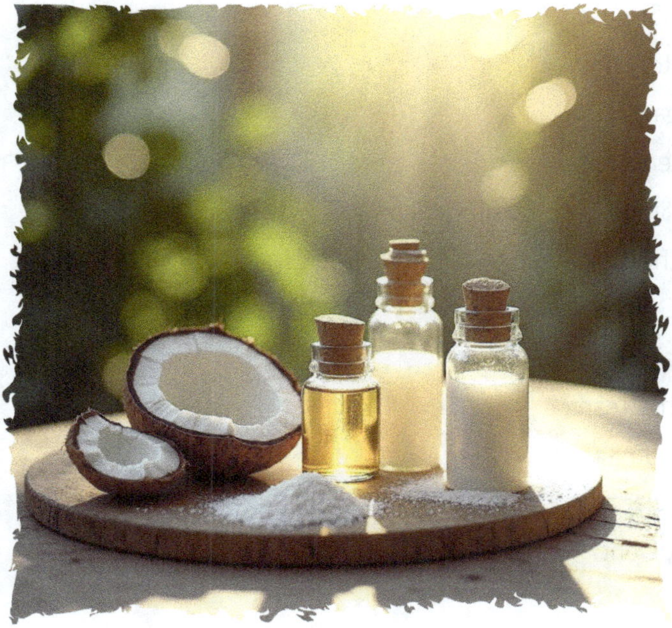

You'll have a product that beats everything sold commercially! For both healthiness and for price. Make sure you tweak it according to your own unique preferences.

Soon your friends will want some. So why not make a larger batch. You might even start your own homemade dentifrice company. There's a nascent market for top-quality niche healing products.

If you choose to go that route, how about some great unique brand names:

1. Starseed Smile.
2. Vitalis Vibe.
3. Luminara Paste.
4. Solara Sparkle.
5. Charmgleam.
6. Vitadentis.
7. ShantiShine.
8. Luzdiente.

9. SanaSonrisa.
10. HaelenMint.
11. Solgard.
12. Phoenix Foam.
13. AséSmile.
14. HózhóWhite.
15. SafiDent.
16. CuraVita.
17. ArohaClean.
18. NuruSmile.
19. Hygieiapaste
20. MinoDent.

The best oral hygiene is the one you design yourself. Having a great homemade dentifrice costs much less and is also much healthier. It puts you ahead of everyone who pays for commercial paste.

And who pays more for commercial paste than the treatment-giver who refuses to see the logic in stress-free care. Until he's convinced, that is....

56

CHAPTER

Shaker 3

A Shakespearean Scene in Ten Relaxing Minutes (just like ART)

Title: The Healing of the Molar

Dramatis Personae:
Dentist (*A steel-wielding traditionalist, speaks in thunderous iambic pentameter*)
Client (*A devotee of Atraumatic Restorative Treatment, speaks in earthy prose*)
Hygienist (*The voice of reason, shifts between verse and prose*)

ACT I, SCENE I

(*The Dentist's lair. The Client sits white-knuckled as the Dentist flourishes a high-speed drill.*)

Dentist: "Behold!
Mine engine of celestial might,
That turns the bleakest caries into light!
With tungsten bit and mercy none,
Fee schedule compensation when I'm done."

Client: (*leaping up*)
"Hold! Thou metal-obsessed brute!
I'll have no part of thy barbaric loot!

Where's ART's kind hand?
The glass ionomer?
The finger tools?
Must all thy cures be terror?"

(*The Hygienist steps between them, clipboard in hand.*)

Hygienist: (*to Dentist*)
"My lord, the times do move.
In fine clinics, I could prove,
Do they heal most dental ills,
with their curettes and honored skills."

ACT I, SCENE II

(*The Client brandishes a*
"Genuine Wellness" pamphlet.)

Client: "See'st thou not?
The future's minimally invasive!
No needles! No noise!
The method's quite persuasive!
We excavate with spoon
and chemic bond,
Then sing lullabies
as oral health responds!"

Dentist: (*clutching drill like Excalibur*)
"Thou spoon-fed heretic!
Dost thou dare scorn
The sacred roar of this,
my cobalt horn?

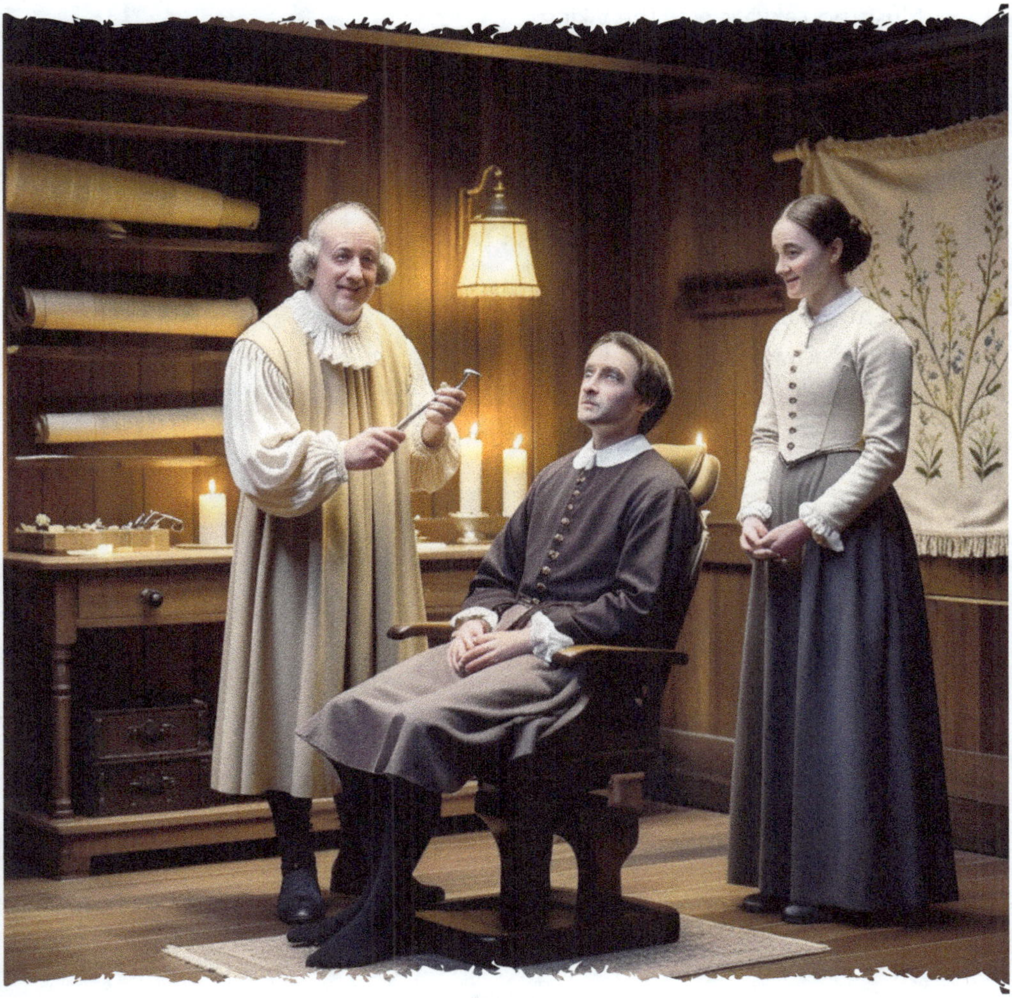

Since Hadrian's day
we've bored to heal -
To shun the bit is treason
to thy enamel's weal!"

(*The Hygienist snatches the drill away. Uneasy silence.*)

Hygienist: "My liege…
the man hath paid upfront in gold!
Must thou always play the Viking,
raiding mouths untold?"

ACT I, SCENE III

(An awakening. The Dentist, newly inspired, mixes glass ionomer cement. The Client nods knowingly.)

Client: "Ha! The lion eats a pear today!
Tell me now, dost thou feel the decay
Of thine own dogma? That drill's but a crutch
For those lacking coursework in atraumatic, much!"

Dentist: (*pauses, then—laughs.*)
"Thanks then, thou whimsical, spoon-trusting sprite.
And mark me, in times to come,
thy teeth shall sing the praises,
of wisdom's clarion light!"

(The Client bows. The Hygienist claps in joy, as the curtain falls.)

FIN

[**note:** the Client's payment in gold is now seen as an overpayment.]

57

CHAPTER

Correctness

Core points:

1. Drilling deeper decay is very high-risk.
2. Caries removal gel doesn't harm sensitive tissues.
3. The vast majority of dentists are unaware of this.

When interviewing dozens of Mexican dentists for the ART treatment, I had a most fascinating encounter.

I asked this dentist about very deep caries. To the pulp layer. I'm insisting on ART only!

Would he insist on drilling if the caries were deep, close to the nerve?

Right away his tune changed!

He said that in such a case, he WON'T drill, but will use the caries removal gel. In Latin American countries it's usually Brix3000, which is made in Argentina.

I was astonished. This drilling dentist won't drill. I asked, "REALLY?"

He explained that so near to the nerve and sensitive pulp, drilling will cause serious trauma, guaranteed. Therefore he won't go near it with the drill.

This dentist is one out of ten thousand (or more?) who correctly understood this serious risk to the tooth's longevity!

I asked, "How do you remove decay?" He replied, "By using a hand tool."

A-HAAA!

This completely CONTRADICTS what nearly all North American dentists will say!

They will say, "We have to use the drill because otherwise, with decay so deep, we won't get it all. We might miss some."

So they're basically saying that it's okay to severely traumatize the pulp and nerve to get ALL the caries out, even the part that is firm and solid.

This is the worst treatment protocol possible.

Using the drill in very deep caries almost guarantees tooth death. Soon, or much sooner than normal.

In such a case, and where tooth longevity is clearly spelled out as an absolute objective, the method MUST be to use a spoon excavator in conjunction with the caries removal gel.

In addition there will likely be a pulp cap, unless GIC (glass ionomer) is used.

THIS and only this is the TOOTH SAVING protocol.

That one Mexican dentist said something few other dentists know. Dentists have no sense of an alternative. They approach the nerve and pulp with a high speed drill because they want to get "everything out".

It's a kind of conditioned response based on a very pervasive college curriculum, which also happens to be quite mistaken.

A dentist logically needs to use a conservative approach, removing only the soft decayed tissue, and leaving the hard viable tissue in place, even if discolored.

The ART method will prove conclusively that tooth survival and longevity are dependent on a clear understanding of the injurious effects of vibration and intense drill-tip heat.

The published studies show that even with water-cooling, the intense heat at the drill-tip is rarely mitigated properly. And this causes severe pulp trauma.

Could the dental college curriculum be so misguided? Has it traded basic common sense for dense layers of ineffective science and technology?

It took one realistic Mexican dentist to validate what every dentist should already know. It's a thunderous realization!

Just so, thunderbolts await healers who are too skilled for their own good. Too good? Well, if you upset the balance of the realms, certain forces take notice...

58

CHAPTER

Thunderbolts

A DRAMA AFTER SOPHOCLES

Title: Trial of Asclepios (Ὕβρις Ἀσκληπιοῦ)

Dramatis Personae:
Zeus: King of Olympus (*Runs the dental boards, voice like thunder, father of Apollo*)
Asclepios: Medical genius (*Sincere, and a bit confused*)
Apollo: Lord of Prophecy and Sunshine. (*Father of Asclepios*)
Hades: Boss of the Underworld (*Zeus's brother*)
Chorus of Olympians: Demiurges and Sprites who comment on the action.

Setting: The great hall of Olympus. A throne of marble. Air thick with tension.

Zeus sits upon his throne, a masterbolt resting against it. Chorus on one side, defendants on the other. Hades opposite, a dark presence amidst the Olympian splendor.

Chorus:

"O bright halls of Olympus, where things have gotten weird,

We've got a nasty family feud, and everyone's got a beard!

Nectar sweet could be this all, above the busy thrall

We do no invasive practice here, dental trauma we forestall.

Dental-based filial discord, it does concern us so!

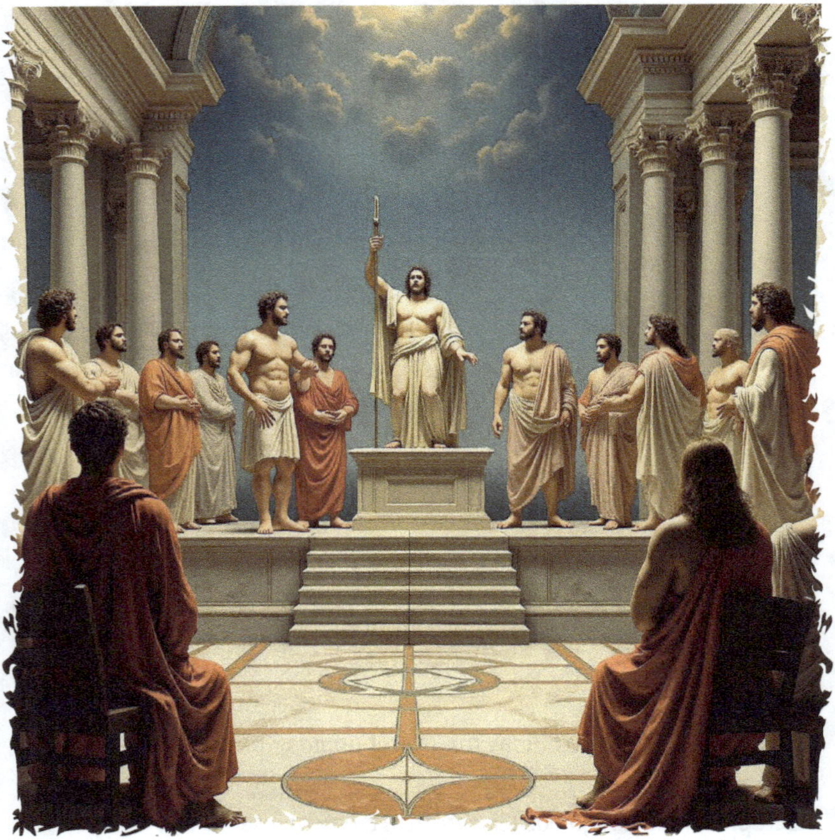

A healer great is accused, for what, we do not know.
The son of Leto's light, bright Apollo, stands,
While from the sunless realm, sullen Hades lands."

Zeus:
"Here sit I, King of Kings
Yet what am I really, then?
Perhaps just a silly blip, on the end of someone's pen?
For without the page, to make me big and strong
I'm but an idea, not knowing where I belong."

Hades: (*Whispers: "Hey, little bro, nice gig!"*)
"Ahem" (*shouts*)
"Great Zeus, we judge a serious crime

That shakes foundational fate and time.
No more do shades with mute acceptance come,
My kingdom echoes with a deafening hum.
The Styxian ferryman finds his manifest thin,
And from the walls of Erebus comes such a din!
Asclepios' evidence-based dental lore,
Has rendered my endodontic horde, mighty sore!"

Zeus: (*Whispers: "No way, bro..."*)
"Ahem..." (*voice thundering*)
"Oh, thou boring and confus'ed scum,
which doth hang out with scoundrel bum.
Bring me some wit, some jovial pun,
Lest it's thee I smite, with 20 megatons."

Apollo: (*steps forth gallantly*)
Defense counsel am I, for my noble son,
Who's done nothing wrong, but sav'ed everyone.
If you do smite him with your thunderbolt,
Your name might be history's stain'ed mote.
Condemn your own grandson, a heinous crime!
And for what cause? But for lucre's shine!"

Zeus:
"Son, this vexes me sore, but what am I to do?
This court, and also pharma, need steady revenue."

Asclepios: (*steps forward boldly*)
"I raised brave Hippolytus, and others, I did too.
CR gel and ozone gas wrought cures they never knew!

So let me once and all, put this wretched trial to rest,
For I've a very bright idea that ranks among the best!"

Zeus:
"Tell me, tell me then. Please don't be shy.
Or you'll hang by your Greek chiton, way up on high."

Asclepios:
"I propose a plan to assuage your optics need;
You shall save face, plus be free of me.
Pretend to smite me, with thunderbolt in hand,
While I shall emigrate to distant Hyperborean lands."

Apollo: (*jumping up and down in glee*)
"He's quite a wit, this healer son of mine!
To charm great Zeus, with solutions so sublime!"

Zeus:
"I'm as great, I suppose, as others make me,
For without the pen, I'd be as a hopping flea.
Asclepios, mind sharp as a cobra's tooth;
I'm shown a victory in appearance, forsooth!
You understand the burdens of the throne.
It is not merely power, but how that power is known!"

Asclepios:

"Then lift your mighty bolt, and do let it roar!
While I slip away forever, through that yonder door!"

Zeus: (*lifts thunderbolt, a mighty boom and flash ensues*)

"The deed is done, and I've restored the dental praxis!
But for how long, as smart mortals flip the axis!"

Apollo:

"They shall flip it soon, for ART'S the light of day!
No longer shall wrong method
rage 'gainst nature's ideal way."

Chorus:

"Aiah! Aiah! The healer is now departed,
Before his work had hardly even started!
A brilliant noble mind, too great for its time,
Has tasted now the fire, of hard Olympian brine.
Join us then again, for litigation yet to come,
As mighty Zeus metes justice, affordably to everyone!"

59

CHAPTER

Capping

Core points:

1. Pulp capping can help save many damaged teeth.
2. Endodontists are far too quick to give up on damaged teeth.
3. A.R.T. has been successfully applied in many severe cases.

"It's too deep. You can't save it! You need a crown!"

WRONG! Bong, Bong, Bong...

We need to arrive at the basics of the restoration of the seriously damaged tooth. It's a requirement, because many people are in that position. Sometimes even because of harmful dentistry!

Once the prep has been done (the decay removal), part two (the restoration) comes in.

You can heal this tooth! Even if the damage is severe. You must try!

You're going to need to listen to your own voice. Not his. That much is obvious!

Pulp capping is a key part of this process. The pulp cap is what's going to keep the sensitive tissue from being harmed by the restoration.

A good pulp cap will definitely help to save that tooth and give it a new life. Maybe even a very long life. That's the outcome we need!

Exposed dental pulp has to be protected. Pulp is a deeper, very sensitive tissue.

When capping, a plastic dycal applicator is used for minimal impact.

There are two kinds of pulp caps: direct and indirect. I'm going to deal here with the direct kind, where the pulp is actually exposed.

It presents a fabulous healing challenge. Why not involve your dentist! Here are some well-inclusive print-outs to show to the dentist:

1. The traditional material is Calcium Hydroxide ($Ca(OH)_2$). It's placed directly over the exposure, then sealed with Glass Ionomer Cement (GIC).
2. Mineral Trioxide Aggregate (MTA) is a newer entry. It's now the gold standard for DPC (direct pulp cap) due to its high success rates (over 95%).
3. Biodentine is similar to MTA but faster setting, and it promotes the formation of new dentin.
4. In ART settings, GIC has been used alone as a pulp cap. It works but has less dentin enhancing ability as the previous two choices.

These are technical points, but are a wake-up call for dentists. GIC is used in ART as the primary filling material. It doesn't require light-curing the way that traditional composite resins do.

ART has a novel approach for deeper caries where pulp is exposed. Rather than drill away all the compromised tissue the way most dentists do, ART protocol allows the firm, stained dentin near the pulp to remain.

The evidence is that this imperfect tissue is healed by the body from the inside. Thus, more vital dental tissue is preserved.

After the pulp cap application, the cavity is sealed with a high-viscosity GIC (Ketac Molar, Fuji IX).

The intention is to minimize the risk of traumatized pulp and dentin. Mechanical drilling would, for certain, produce damaging trauma to these sensitive tissues.

In all ART pulp capping, you're most likely saving a valuable tooth that's been given up on by most dentists!

Dentistry is incredibly quick to give up on teeth, recommending root canals, even though the tooth might be quite viable!

Dentists, as I've mentioned several times now, are not especially well-trained in dental longevity. Their repair methods are meant to be convenient. For whom? For them, of course!

It's the deep caries into the pulp layer that does it every time. Such teeth can and must be saved. And it's not hard with pulp capping and minimal excavation of viable but compromised tissue.

Of course, the drill renders this nuance almost impossible. The drill-wielding dentist will see the task as impossible.

When capping pulp exposed teeth, only very biocompatible material is used. It builds up the tissue to form what's known as "secondary dentin".

If your dentist is unaware of this vital tooth-saving method, it's best to print the following for his benefit:

1. MTA (Mineral Trioxide Aggregate) is the best.
2. Use Angelus fast-set pre-mixed MTA. It's biocompatible, it's very effective at sealing, and it's less technique sensitive than the calcium hydroxide (which makes it excellent for ART-trained hygienists).
3. Biodentine is expensive but it's an excellent second choice. It's easy to work with and sets quickly.

Your dentist will appreciate this very much. It adds a strong dental-longevity capability to his skill-set.

In pulp capping the best ART tools are spoon excavators (with the CR gel for caries removal), disposable ART excavators, and dycal applicators.

The plastic tool is much better than metal in this case. You'll need to tell the dentist. Otherwise he just won't know.

He'll want to jump into a root canal procedure because it's the only thing he's ever been taught about deep caries situations! 100% wrong, of course.

If this feels a bit technical, no problem. You now know a lot more about saving good teeth than much of the dental college curriculum!

That's either amazing or sad, depending how you view it. Either way, dental healing is always seriously good news!

Are we ready for some miracles? Hold on! These accounts need to be covered in depth in the dental curriculum.

If they're not, then we know where their priorities lie!

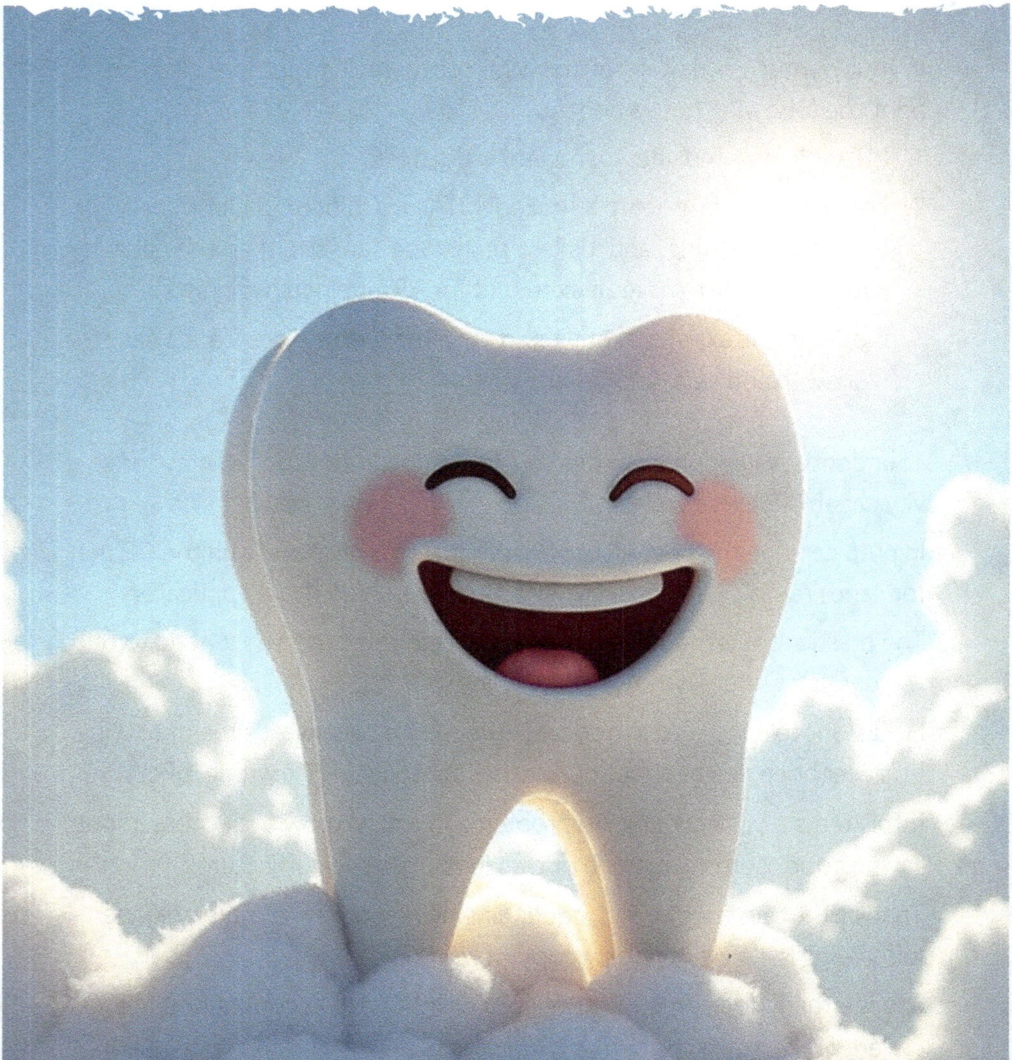

60

CHAPTER

Miracle Saves

Core points:

1. A saved tooth could become completely functional.
2. Severe damage can be reversed.
3. Commercial dentistry requires a healing approach.

In deep dental lore, there are legends of amazing successes in restoring teeth to optimal condition. Why don't we hear about these amazing solutions?

We have some recent evidence of remarkable dental treatment successes.

Case 1: a deep decay pulp-cap success.

A #30 lower right molar had deep caries touching pulp. The dentist (true to standard protocol) recommended RCT (root canal) and crown.

The drill-free solution was to apply Carosolv gel (15 minutes), ART scraping to cleanse all non-viable tissue, application of a Biodentine pulp-cap, and a GIC (glass ionomer Fuji IX) restoration.

Outcome: Five year follow-up, no symptoms, vital pulp, living tooth. Study author: Taha, 2018.

Case 2: a cracked molar, fiber-splint save.

A #14 upper-left molar had a vertical crack. The dentist's standard protocol called for extraction and an implant.

The drill-free solution was to use a Ribbond fiber-splint (bonded across the crack), and a bioceramic sealer (Ceraseal).

Outcome: Seven-year follow-up showed normal function and no pain. Study author: Signore, 2021.

Case 3: a necrotic pulp revascularization.

A #9 upper front tooth had trauma-induced necrosis. Dental standard protocol said "non-vital, hopeless, requires implant".

The drill-free solution was to use Er-YAG laser disinfection, and a PRF (platelet-rich fibrin) deep application to regenerate the pulp.

Outcome: Pulp vitality restored within 12 months. Functioning tooth. Study author: Jung, 2018.

Case 4: a failed amalgam glass-hybrid repair.

A #19 lower left molar had recurring decay under an old amalgam. Dental protocol said "We placed a toxic mercury amalgam, but now you need to pay us again to remove it".

The drill-free solution was to use specialized hand-tools only to remove the amalgam, then a EQUIA Forta glass-hybrid restoration.

Outcome: At 8 years, no secondary decay and a viable living tooth. (Regular dentistry still insisted on being fully paid to fix their own mistakes.) Study author: Mickenautsch, 2020.

References include: an IAOMT 2023 paper titled "Biomimetic Protocols for Complex Cases", and a Jo Frencken 2018 paper titled "ART Success".

It is no understatement to say that these are miracle cases. But at the same time, these cures SHOULD be the normal way of doing things.

The fact that they're not explains everything you need to know about the modern BUSINESS of dentistry.

If we want good healing dentistry, we will need to be our own bosses when it comes to our teeth. There's no way around it.

We can try changing the entire structure of dentistry, but then we'd have to decouple the commercial industry from the profession and from all its boards and curriculum designers. Doing this would require an actionable force.

On the other hand, we can simply empower ourselves with the kind of keen knowledge that takes all the fake mystery out of dental wellness.

Teeth are basically simple. They want to be optimally fit and well. Common sense wins every time!

Now we're going to have to convince "the trade" about what we really want. It's different now. We're never going back to that injurious method.

61

CHAPTER

No-Compromise *Letter*

Core points:

1. Approach every dentist on your own terms.
2. Engage directly, not via a receptionist.
3. Be 100% clear on your goals.

Starting out in looking for ART-only treatment, things might be intimidating for you. If you're asking a regular dentist, it won't be easy.

To deliver better odds of success, here is a no-compromise request letter to make your objectives crystal clear to everyone:

Dear Dr.

I hereby request the safest possible dental treatment. My teeth are seriously close friends of mine!

My basic objective is tooth longevity. That's where my teeth and I stick together for a very long time! Relax. This might be a new concept for you!

High-speed drilling is a nasty business for teeth. Just ask the tooth fairy! Hand instruments only for me, buddy!

I also brought evidence:

Zach & Cohen (1965): 5.5°C temperature rise causes pulp necrosis.

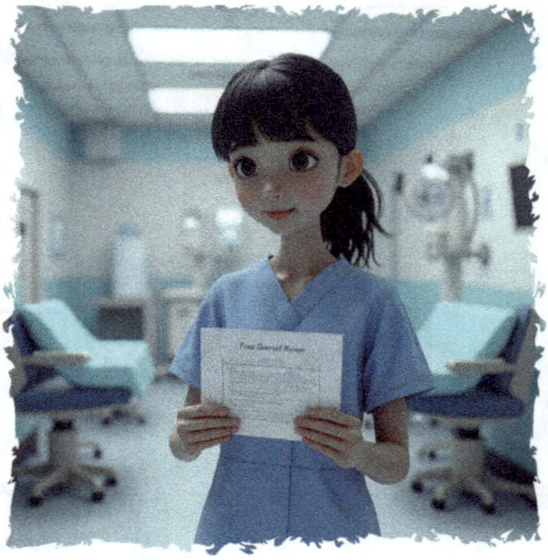

Brännström (1960s–80s): Drill vibration creates microcracks, the beginning of the end!

Banerjee (2000): 72% of drilled teeth develop subsurface fractures. Say it ain't so, buddy!

The solution is very ART-istic, buddy! Are you on board yet?

All right, you performed 500 drill procedures in college. I'm here to suggest some serious re-edumacation.

This latte is getting cold. So say it! Yes or no?

Failed restorations make for a very lousy afternoon. So does needless pain.

That needle ain't my buddy, buddy. Get it out of my sight. I reject all rotary instruments. This is fancy for "drill".

I shall insist on:

1. Hand excavators.
2. Caries removal gel.
3. Glass ionomer restoration.

If you don't whip that dental healing arse in gear, I shall take my wad of dough elsewhere!

Or, maybe I'm just going to convert you. Right now!

Sincerely,

Notary Seal (for added emphasis):

This letter really bangs! Make sure to tailor it to your own style.

A good investigation often yields amazing results. Why not check in on the greatest investigator of all? His rooms are the epitome of cozy elegance. Plus, he's fooled by nothing!

62

CHAPTER

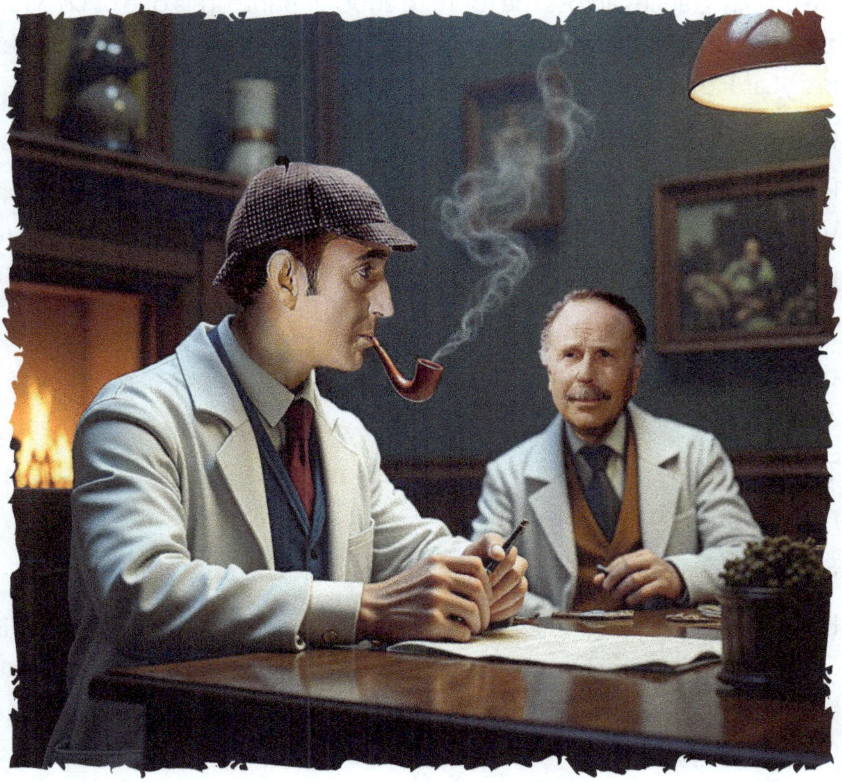

Holmes 2

Scene: 221B Baker Street,
the Holmes Dental Healing Spa.

Holmes is relaxing in front of the fireplace, puffing blissful clouds of his choicest Oriental shag blend while carefully studying a telegram scrip that arrived five minutes earlier.

The window is open. Watson studies him carefully, then his gaze moves to the wall, where Holmes' dental college graduation group portrait hangs. He gets up and walks to it, and winces uncomfortably.

He quickly glances across the room to another photo, this one of Dr. Salazar Stevens, a classmate, with an industry medallion for most crown sales in a year. He shrugs and shakes his head with imperceptible cynicism.

Holmes: "You're entirely correct, Watson! Invasive dentistry has a most peculiar reward chain!"

Watson: (with a start) "Upon my word, Holmes! How could you possibly know..."

Holmes: (interrupting) "Elementary, Watson..." (he tosses the note into the fire) "...And if I'm not mistaken, our detractor is about to pay us a visit at any time now..."

The door chime rings from below. In a few moments, Mrs. Hudson is ushering Stevens into the Spa.

Stevens: (snatching up a vial, sneering) "What's this jelly, Holmes?"

Holmes: (calmly retrieves the vial) "Handle with care, Stevens. This 'jelly' simply represents the curative future. It's Carisolv. Or rather, the active principle derived from a far more accessible source: the humble Carica papaya."

Watson: (eagerly) "It's remarkable, Stevens! The papain enzyme specifically targets denatured collagen in carious dentin. It softens the caries with astonishing precision..."

Stevens: (barking a laugh) "Papaya? Too good to be true! Where is the anxiety?"

Holmes: (holding the vial to the light) "Exactly, Stevens. Observe the elegance as I apply the gel to this typodont. Wait moments. Gently lift the soft denatured dentin away with a hand instrument. No excavation of healthy tooth structure. No searing heat. No harmful vibration. Completely painless and so, usually needle-free. The patient feels nothing, save, of course, immense relief."

Stevens: "Painless? And you plan to fundamentally improve dentistry?"

Holmes: "This gel, Stevens, is direct in its specificity. It targets only the substrate. As for sterility, the formulation is impeccable. As for technology, harnessing natural enzymatic action is the pinnacle of biochemical engineering."

Watson: "And the cost, Stevens! A fraction of high-speed drills, burs, and air compressors! Not to mention the trauma and discomfort that would be negated at last. Patients everywhere, rejoicing!"

Stevens: "In a profit-based industry, there are regulatory boards to impede such breakthroughs, Holmes."

Holmes: "Stevens, wonderful cures like this one should be better available. And if not, do tell me why."

Stevens: "It's obvious, Holmes! The support structures of a business profession dislike alternate curatives. Especially when very inexpensive."

Watson: "My word, Stevens. You seem to be veering inexorably towards the truth!"

Holmes: "Let him continue, Watson. This may be a new Stevens. I fancy his episode from last week may have had a beneficial effect."

Stevens: "You've forced me into a corner Holmes! I always saw you as a bright student. I didn't understand your purposes. Now, I think I finally do…"

Holmes: "And in a good way?"

Stevens: "You shall be famous, Holmes. Mark my words. You want nothing less than to relieve the needless suffering of millions."

Watson: "A new Stevens…"

Stevens: "Holmes, I cannot say how kind the boards and the regulators will be towards your methods. But I will say this. The public will appreciate this immensely."

Holmes: "Salazar. You're still the same reckless eager student you were so many years ago. Except that now… you're human! I say this kindly, of course."

Stevens: "Holmes, Watson. We build a new bridge. So many repairs on the old one. So we make a new one."

Holmes: "Stevens, Mrs. Hudson brews a wonderful pot of tea! And we happen to have a cup here with your name on it!"

63

CHAPTER

Iatrogenic Realities

Core points:

1. Commercial dentistry has been called "a disaster".
2. Deep anger remains from harms done.
3. Money's Worth is an active principle.
4. People expect to be miserable in dental treatment, and it's a fundamental fallacy.

Medical injury is called iatrogenic. It's been a great concern to many.

The philosopher Leibniz felt that the established medicine was potentially dangerous.

Huang-Ti, the Yellow Emperor of China, wanted to design a medicine that was ideal. The missing Wei Jing probably carries a treasure-house of practical knowledge.

Dentistry, for most people, is anything but fun! People "grin and bear it". Is this necessary? Absolutely not!

Dentistry must become FUN! ART is the foundation! Sincerity is the FUEL!

The solution to miserable dentistry is NOT more smile marketing, it's delivering genuine safety and value! Radical concepts!

There is a book called "Cure Tooth Decay" by Ramiel Nagel which makes an impassioned jeremiad. The allegations are really startling:

1. "Modern dentistry is a profound failure. The enormity of suffering and disease caused by dentistry is so massive that it is beyond comprehension."

Uh-oh. The author experienced great disappointment in his dental treatments. He doesn't say a lot of suffering, he says "massive."

Is it really beyond comprehension? Dentistry is a core profession, a core service! How could it be such a "profound failure"? What happened? And for how long has this gone on?

2. "Its treatment methods of drilling and filling are highly damaging to teeth."

Yes, this is documented in the many studies referenced here. Sources are listed in the back pages.

3. "The materials used in dentistry are extremely toxic and have been connected to diseases that are severe, painful and widespread."

What kind of toxins? Perhaps anesthesia? Has it been contaminated? Have there been lab tests to find out?

This matters because the very definition of "iatrogenic" involves an issue like this.

4. "Conventional dentistry has placed highly poisonous mercury in the mouths of hundreds of millions of people."

Yes, this is spot on. Mercury is gradually being phased out because "the public finally knows".

5. "Tens of millions of needless root canals have been performed."

Root canals are a regular practice. It's true that the vast majority of them are needless. The tooth becomes a prosthetic.

6. "Modern dentistry has drilled deeply into healthy parts of millions of teeth because of the failed treatment policy of "extension for prevention."

This relates not just to "anchoring" of very toxic fillings (sometimes resulting in hospitalizations) but also to removal of healthy tissues for "ease of work". It's the very essence of iatrogenesis.

7. "It has caused irreversible pulp damage in millions of tooth nerves with drills that spin too fast."

The pulp damage leads to tooth loss.

8. "The profit-motivated system of dentistry has led to tens of millions of needless dental procedures."

Profit-motivation doesn't automatically need to lead to dire results. Incentives need to be created to reward excellent healing craft.

9. "If this dental massacre had any benefits to show then perhaps it could be exonerated. But it does not."

Is it really a "massacre"? This writer had difficult experiences in dentistry. How many people are in the same boat?

There are reputable studies looking at the "discomfort of the dental experience".

A top one is Abrahamsson's 2017 paper called "Dental Anxiety and Experiences of Negative Dental Treatment for Dental Avoidance".

It said:

"Phobic dental avoidance is related to anticipatory stress and anxiety reactions, negative oral health effects, and psychological distress."

There it is! People EXPECT pain and discomfort with dentistry!

And unless you're Eeyore, the A.A. Milne donkey, you don't want any part of this!

You want comfortable, pain-free dental treatment!

And you might have thought it was impossible to find such a thing!

Then... you found a magic book!

Way up in Russia, a big time CEO had a traumatic epiphany, and the outcome was most positive...

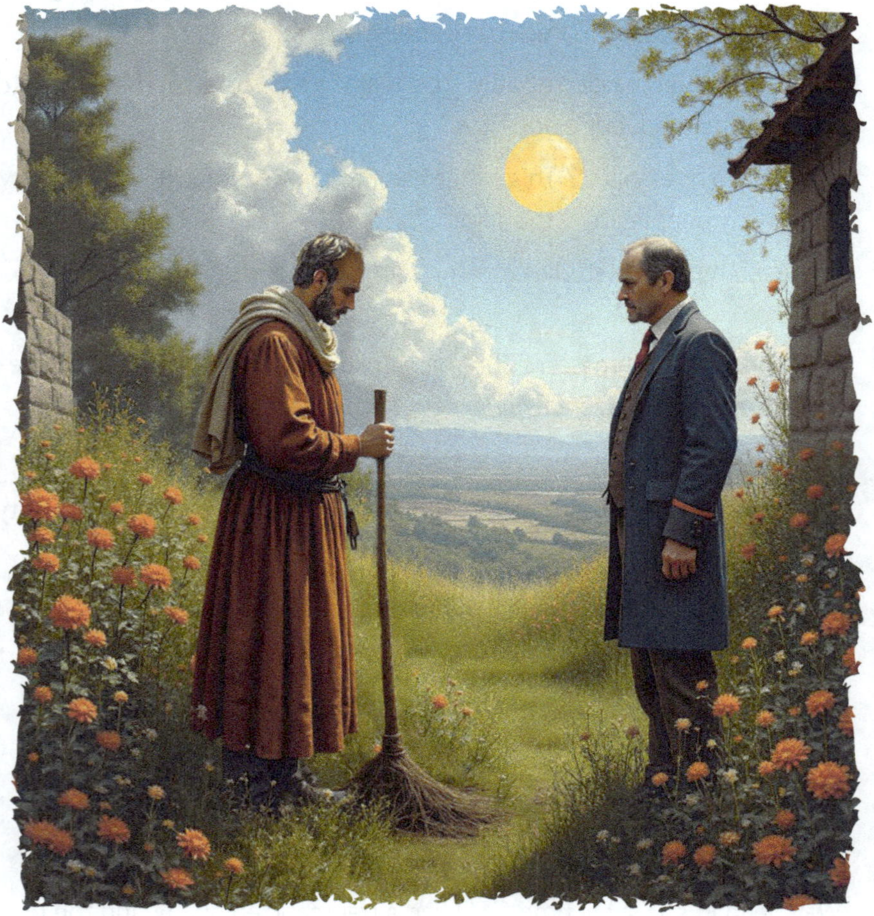

64

CHAPTER

Dacha

Fyodor Dostoevsky's boardroom breakdown story was graphic. Now we're far outside the city, in a peaceful corner of the countryside.

The late summer sun gilds the birch trees lining the dirt track to Pyotr Volkov's dacha. (*The dacha is the classic Russian countryside cottage, often hosting an abundant orchard and garden*).

Bees drone over lavender. Pyotr (*60s, weathered face, simple clothes, hands stained with earth*) kneels amongst raised beds of chamomile and mint. His days as Zenith Pharma CEO are far behind him. Or?

A sleek black Mercedes hums to a halt, kicking up dust. Dmitri Sokolov (*CFO, sharp suit, uneasy*) and Anya Petrova (*Head of Marketing, immaculate, scanning the scene with disdain*) emerge.

Anya: (*forcing brightness*) "Pyotr Alexeyevich! Such rustic serenity! Though, honestly… one worries for the suspension."

Pyotr wipes hands on his trousers, and stands slowly.

Pyotr: "Dmitri. Anya. Didn't expect… auditors. Tea? Mint's fresh. Or comfrey, for overall radiance."

Dmitri: (*clears throat*) "No tea, Pyotr. We're here on business. Serious business. Zenith needs you. Badly."

Pyotr: "Zenith? Sold my shares. Paid for these cabbages. And the cozy cottage…"

Anya: (*scoffs lightly*) "Cabbages! Pyotr, be serious. You built Zenith. That instinct… that vision… it doesn't just vanish because you've taken up… gardening. Xylozap generics are looming. The sharks circle…"

Dmitri: "The board is panicking. Weak leadership. They need your steady hand. Your understanding of the… levers. Come back as Senior Advisor. Name your price. Seven figures. Eight. Whatever it takes."

Pyotr picks a ripe raspberry, and offers it. They decline.

Pyotr: "Price? You still talk only in price, Dmitri. What's the price of clean earth under your nails? The price of sunlight on basil?"

Anya: (*impatient*) "Poetic, Pyotr, truly. But this is reality. Millions of patients rely on Zenith! Without strong leadership, innovation stalls! Shareholders file actions!"

Pyotr: (*quietly intense*) "Lives? Like the lives impacted by suppressing the Siberian Hericium mushroom? The ones who paid with everything for Xylozap while a forest cure grew wild? You remember that lever, Anya? The suppression lever?"

Dmitri: (*flustered*) "Ancient history! Regulatory necessities! We're talking about the future! Zenith's future! Your legacy!"

Pyotr: "My legacy? This is my legacy now." (*gestures to the thriving garden*) "Real things. Things that grow, heal, feed… without patents, without fear campaigns, without filtering out 'non-viable demographics'. Simple. True."

Anya: (*voice hardening*) "Don't be naïve. The world runs on the game. On winning. You were the best at it. This… (*waves a manicured hand dismissively*)… is surrender. Playing peasant while the real game goes on."

Pyotr: (*a sad smile*) "Surrender? No, Anya. It's the only victory I ever truly won. Escaping the ledger."

Dmitri: "Ledger? What ledger? The balance sheets are solid! For now! We need you!"

Pyotr: "Not your ledger, Dmitri. The other one. The one weighed in destiny, not rubles. The one I saw tip… in that boardroom. I'm balancing mine. Here. With dirt and seeds and quiet. You couldn't pay me enough to go back into debt on that scale. Not with all the gold in Zurich."

Anya: (*scoffs, turns away*) "Madness. The stress broke him after all, Dmitri. Wasted trip. Let's go. The stench of manure is… overwhelming."

Dmitri: (*desperate, steps closer*)

"Pyotr, think! The power! The influence! You're throwing it away for… weeds!"

Pyotr: (*looks past them, to the birches*) "Not weeds, Dmitri. Freedom. Things your spreadsheets can't quantify. Things your black car can't carry you to. Go back to your game. Play it well…"

Anya: (*already heading to the car*) "Come, Dmitri. We have actual strategists to see. Enjoy your… cabbages, Pyotr."

Dmitri hesitates, looks at Pyotr's calm, earth-stained face, then follows Anya. The Mercedes door slams. The engine growls, then fades down the dusty track.

Pyotr kneels back in the soil. He presses his palm flat against the warm, living earth. A bee lands on his sleeve. He smiles faintly, a deep, quiet resignation to his path.

65

CHAPTER

Success

Core points:

1. Dental success is huge in overall wellness.
2. Success is a creative process.
3. Horse traders prioritize the teeth as indicators of overall fitness.

Success is a magic word that has many meanings, as people improve the definition.

When my success also becomes your success, we're onto a good thing!

One thing we mostly agree on is that a good word brings an energy of wanting to find better meanings. Soon the good energy is the thing, not so much the word.

A great domain name can be a lot of fun. Someone with a domain name like "x.com" might really go places with it! Even to Mars? Anything's possible!

A name like "dentalhealer.com" is also cool, albeit a bit longer. Now we have to live up to it! That's the fun!

Same with success. There is a book about almost always being in the present moment. It's a very obscure book (found only in musty used bookshops with squeaky wooden floors and a very large cat perched on a shelf) and it's called "The Power of Pretty Darn Soon".

This is a truly powerful book. One realizes that "pretty soon" opens up a world of opportunities. Much stronger than having your face on the screen of the "right now", so to speak.

With "pretty darn soon" you have the luxury of time. You get to breathe. You're not urgent all the time.

The ultimate aficionado of "pretty darn soon" is Winnie the Pooh. The Pooh bear specialized in putting off until tomorrow (or later) what didn't absolutely need to be done today. He banked time! That's power.

Time seems to be like a river of energy. It's flowing by you all the time, and you don't really notice it unless you stop and look at a clock.

If you're feeling great, having fun, it seems to zip by.

Upstream is the future. It hasn't reached you yet. Downstream is the past. You read the history of it. It's flowed by you already.

If you're able to look upstream at what's coming, that makes you a prophet. It's a good gig if you're really up for it.

Mind you, being able to discern next week's winning lotto numbers requires a really sharp telescope. Not many prophets can do that.

But if you could, you'd obviously be super-successful. The trick with time, then, is to let it run its course and try to worry over it as little as possible. Then, you're like the Pooh bear. You're on top of things.

So we think about what the wise ones said about success. Then we remember: "Seek first the greater, along with the righteousness, and the lesser will be added also."

Wow. We step back. We'll get the greater that we seek, but ALSO the lesser? Could this be true?

This changes things. The greater and the lesser also! Almost like a healthy dental treatment AND no discomfort in the process!

And righteousness is the magic sauce that makes it all happen! Now it all makes sense!

Admittedly, many seek gold. That's because gold has been a facsimile store of value since ancient times. When paper money goes up and down (usually down) they turn to gold.

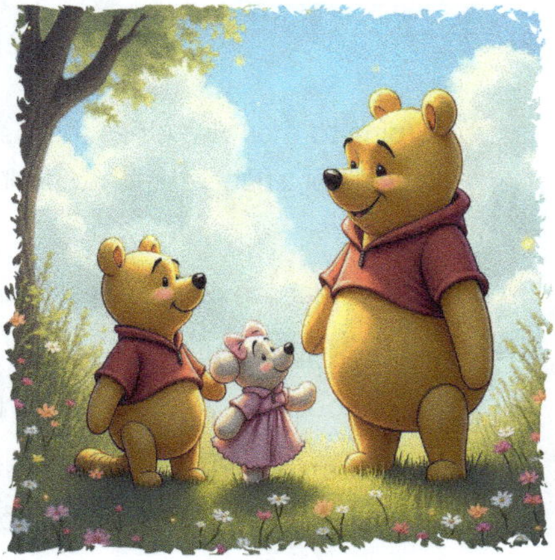

So what could be greater than gold? Ah, more brutal questions! Things greater than gold! That shiny metal that's been valued by royalty and pauper alike.

Obviously the ability to enjoy that gold must be greater!

Yes, we must ask! In the asking is the finding! With a process of discovery wedged between.

Concentrated capital might be a powerful thing. It turns the Golden Rule on its head. It also likes safe harbors.

If you were a horse trader, and you were considering a nice specimen to purchase, chances are, you'd make a beeline for the teeth.

That's what horse traders do. They check the teeth first. Then they know if they have a good horse or not.

Often they have an all-right horse, which might even talk like a person after being given peanut butter, the way Mr. Ed did.

Mr. Ed was one serious horse. The wisdom of a Socrates. Few horses are like that. Alas, it was a television horse. He sold consumer products. Someone's homemade dentifrice perhaps?

Focal Theory explains that an issue in oral health might manifest as a symptom in a totally different part of the body. Like toxic fillings causing a malady elsewhere.

Medicine cannot always make the connection because doctors are discouraged from examining teeth!

That might be a good thing, depending on the doctor. Luckily I don't own "medicine.com". Too much responsibility. A coach has to focus!

According to the Wise Ones then, success is the single-minded, prioritized pursuit of a right relationship with the Creative Essence, the One who lives forever.

Trusting in that provision is trusting in the correctness of the process.

So we keep asking what the greater meaning of success is, knowing that with righteousness, we'd obtain the lesser as well.

A word is a solidified form of an idea, which is often about a worthy desire. Desires are good! It's the yearning for better things!

The energy behind a word and an idea gives it power, so we define that energy better. We look for it. And we get some powerful refrigerator magnet content!

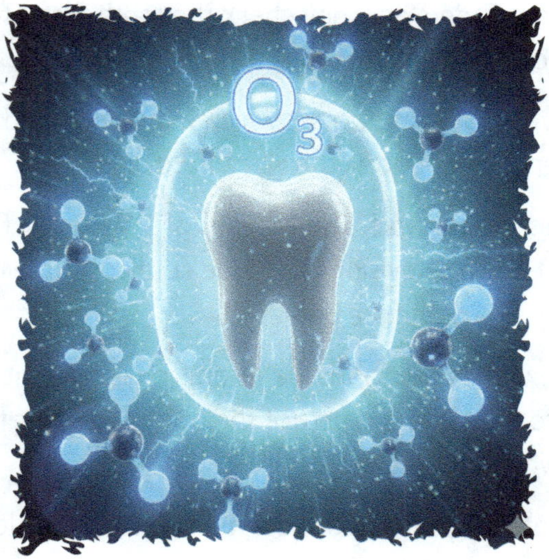

66

CHAPTER

Oxygen

Core points:

1. Pure ozone is a powerful aid in dentistry.
2. It is nearly 100% effective with no side effects.
3. All root canals require regular ozonation.

For the most serious dental healing, there's a protocol that combines ART with ozone. Buckle up. We're in some rare territory here!

What is ozone? It's actually pure oxygen, with an extra atom. It's written as O_3. It's really super-healing.

Athletes know all about hyperbaric oxygen chambers, where they can a ccelerate the healing process.

They need to get back on the playing field. Someone is paying them millions to play, not sit!

A study by Huth blew the game open with regard to healing necrotic teeth. Necrotic means, for all intents and purposes, dead. Teeth that are considered beyond all hope.

Stop right there. Not so, said Huth.

Huth is a great Star Wars name. Like a grim Jedi colonel on a remote icy outpost. And like that forgotten place are teeth that have been given up on.

Huth rewrote the entire endodontics game-board, which is about root canals.

The study is called "Efficacy of Ozone and Platelet-Rich Fibrin in Pulp Revascularization of Necrotic Teeth".

That's a long title all right. But not as long as the wait for a new living tooth once your beloved tooth has become a prosthetic.

The following is a bit technical, but underneath is truth and elegance.

The ART-based ozone disinfection phase:

1. Hand tools only (no rotary files).
2. Ozone insufflation: (60 seconds at 55 μg/mL.
3. Penetrates dentin tubules and lateral canals.
4. Ozonated saline irrigation (2 minutes to flush debris)
5. PRF (Platelet-Rich Fibrin) injection (into canal space, stimulating stem cell migration)
6. Bioceramic coronal seal. (Biodentine placed over PRF to prevent microleakage).

This is the technical process to save a tooth that was given up on.

Combining this with the ART protocol will yield miracles, for sure. There are specialists in ozone treatment. They will understand all of this readily.

The results:

1. Pulp revascularization (74% at 18 months).
2. Apical lesion healing (89%).
3. Dentin wall thickening (68%).

This is technical language for excellent results! Here are some key findings:

1. Ozone gave 99% bacterial reduction.
2. PRF regenerated pulp-like tissue. (histology confirmed vascularization).
3. Teeth retained vitality.

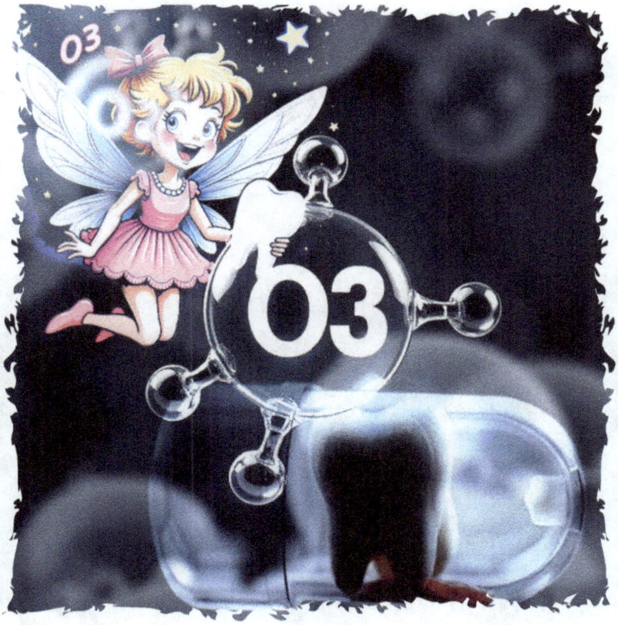

In dental college education, the dogma is that necrotic pulp equals RCT (root canal). In fact, often much less equals the RCT!

We might justifiably say that "professional laziness equals an RCT".

The "ADA Guidelines" that steer the industry still classify ozone as "alternative", despite over 1,200 studies proving its efficacy. It's business, folks.

Oxygen is truly a wonder and a miracle. It's such a potent healer and disinfectant.

Why don't all those glossy dental journals embrace it? How about the widely-lecturing Dr. Horace Drillbit DDS, adjunct professor of endodontic excellence, and his fifteen staff members.

Lucky that WE know about it! Also lucky is how we get to prepare all our encounters with the profession with a strong stance on exactly what we're seeking.

For example, a more urgent sounding letter...

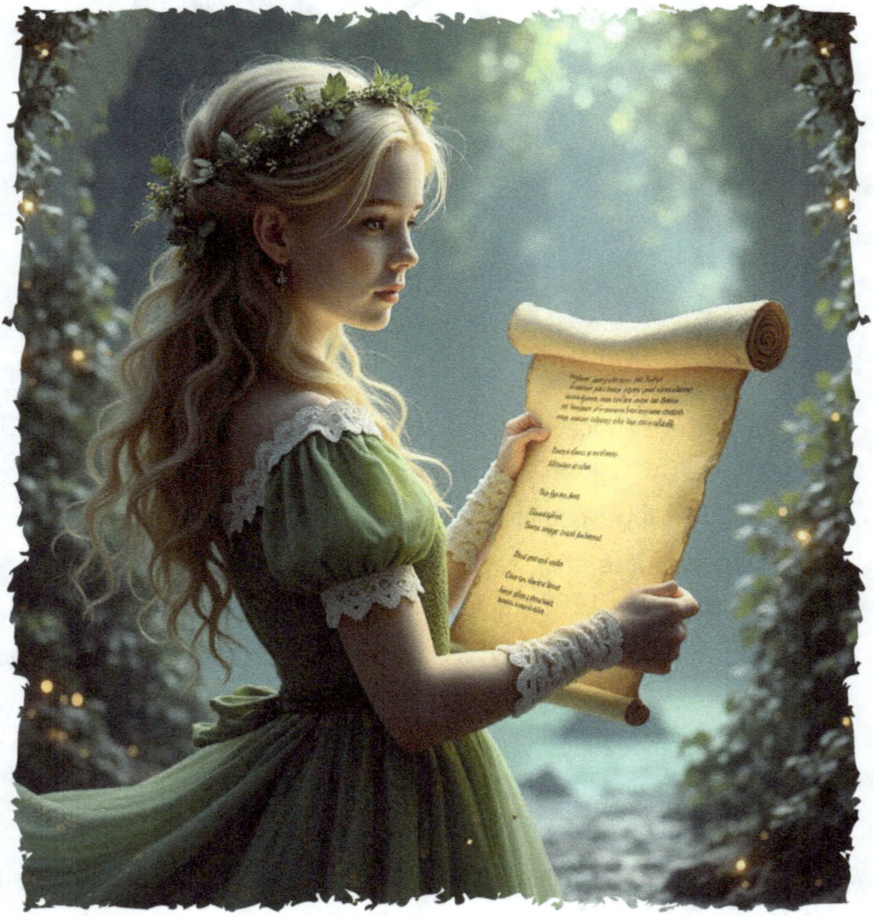

67

CHAPTER

A Defensive *Script*

Core points:

1. Tooth-saving protocols to avoid a "terminal treatment" (RCT).
2. Insisting on the correct way is empowering.

We're getting a large sheet of bright yellow paper. We have strong words to bring to the party!

If you're in a dental crisis where a root canal or implant is the only given diagnosis, do step back. These treatments are irreversible, so we have to save that tooth!

Strong action is needed as there's no room for error. A well-worded script will turn the tables!

"Dear Dental Wellness Provider,

I'm very sorry, but this tooth went to pot. Yes, I know. It's injured and you're calling it necrotic and in need of a root canal procedure. Except that we can save this tooth, and by golly we will!

I held a wedding ceremony last night and I legally married this tooth! Do you know what "through thick and through thin" is? It means we save it!

You don't know Huth but in 2021, he made a big-time rescue protocol. It goes like this:

1. Ozone disinfection (gas + saline)
2. PRF injection
3. Bioceramic seal (Biodentine)

Bottom line: I refuse the traditional root canal treatment (RCT). Are you hoppin' yet? It's right here:

1. 80% of RCTs can be avoided by using the ozone / PRF protocol.
2. Ozone eliminates residual bacteria missed by hand excavation.
3. It stimulates remineralization by oxidizing biofilm and increasing local oxygen.
4. There's no pulp irritation (unlike antiseptics like chlorhexidine).
5. Ozone reduces the need for any aggressive removal (40% less dentin loss).
6. It reduces bacteria by 99.9%.
7. Ozone treatments produce 50% thicker reparative dentin.
8. Ozone breaks down the "EPS matrix" of caries-causing biofilms.
9. The ozone ensures sterile dentin before sealing. It promotes faster healing.
10. Ozone upregulates "pulp stem cells" (accelerates tertiary dentin formation).
11. Even deep caries can be treated with near-zero pulp exposure, eliminating the risk of drilling.

Do you feel like a freshman student again? My alter-ego is "greatest tooth saver of all time"! I'm close personal friends with the Tooth Fairy. You must LISTEN!

I will make it simple for you:

1. Hand tools and caries removal gel are used to prepare the restoration.
2. Ozone is applied for 10 to 30 seconds to sterilize the cavity (no leftover bacteria).
3. The tooth is sealed with a bioactive GIC filling (no drilling needed).

You did four years! You never met the Tooth Fairy yet! Get on it!

We're going to save this tooth because I do not divorce those with whom I feel very close!

Sincerely,

Adjust this script as needed. It's about dental longevity!

Ozone machines can be purchased online. The Chinese are making them for under 2000$. Of course they are! They make everything except ambient lofi chillout. Wait. They make that too.

Ozone penetrates the tiny tubules in dentin. If anyone has root canals, regular ozonation is a must!

For deep cavities, ozone and ART has a 91 % success rate. This is a phenomenal number.

A 2016 Baysan study showed zero pulpitis (severe pulp inflammation) after regular ozone was used.

An ART with ozone treatment has no needles and no drill. It almost rewrites reality itself.

A saved tooth is a living tooth. Just make sure to ozonate any existing root canals often!

A good script bangs! Don't be shy. Insist on what's right.

68

CHAPTER

Ayurveda

Core points:

1. Modern healthcare has much to learn from ancient knowledge.
2. Plant-based curatives often have no side effects.

"Life is fundamentally a field of intelligence and pure knowledge."

This is according to the Charaka Samhita, a book on Ayurvedic medicine.

A deep study by Purohit and Singh focused on Ayurvedic dental health. Here's a condensed summary:

1. Plant-based medicines come from roots, leaves, fruits, barks and seeds.
2. Being patent-free, they're often cheap and effective with minimal si-de-effects.
3. The mizwak stick (Salvadora persica) is a twig from the Arak (Peelu) tree.
4. It works as a toothbrush after the end is frayed. The fibers release silica and tannins to reduce cavities and plaque.
5. Mizwak is anti-bacterial in a very natural way. Its use is ancient.
6. Most Arabian countries plus much of Africa uses mizwaks.
7. The Neem tree is also a "toothbrush tree" from India. Neem makes an excellent healing oil.
8. Neem was tested vs. commercial toothpastes and came out ahead for removing plaque effectively.
9. Oil pulling is done by swishing one or two tablespoons of a good organic oil, such as sesame, coconut, olive, or sunflower.

10. Swish for 15 to 25 minutes (best on an empty stomach) and then spit it out.
11. Organic, unrefined, cold pressed oils contain the best essence.
12. Oil pulling cures many systemic maladies and solves foul breath issues.
13. Amla is the "Indian gooseberry", a vitamin C powerhouse and an astringent.
14. It promotes longevity and induces nourishment.
15. The Charaka Samhita says "it deserves every praise, as it counteracts aging".
16. It also "imparts strength to the intellect and the senses."
17. Bilberry fruit (Vaccinium Myrtillus) and Hawthorn berry (Crateagus Oxycanthus) stabilize collagen, strengthening gum tissue.
18. Bilberry is a natural vision-improver. Pilots used bilberry chutneys as it helped them fly safely for longer.
19. Licorice root (Glycyrrhiza Glabral) reduces plaque, caries, and bacteria.
20. In south India, mango leaf is chewed for cleaning teeth.
21. Mangiferin is a strongly antibacterial compound present in mango leaves.
22. An indoor mango tree would be a great addition as a dental healing house plant.
23. Yellow dock root, alfalfa leaf, cinnamon bark, pomegranate peel, and turmeric root are all highly-regarded dental medicinals.
24. Turmeric (Curcuma longa) heals many gum issues.
25. Clove (Syzygium aromaticum) is a eugenol-rich natural anesthetic/antiseptic for pain relief.

On the warning side, Singh and Purohit mention that "50% of commercial drugs have serious adverse effects not detected prior to their approval."

This is a serious charge! You won't find these problems at the Luminara Dental Healing Spa!

Why? Because the Tooth Fairy has officially approved it. In fact, she might even be running the reception desk!

Meanwhile, a movie set is raising some big noise!

69

CHAPTER

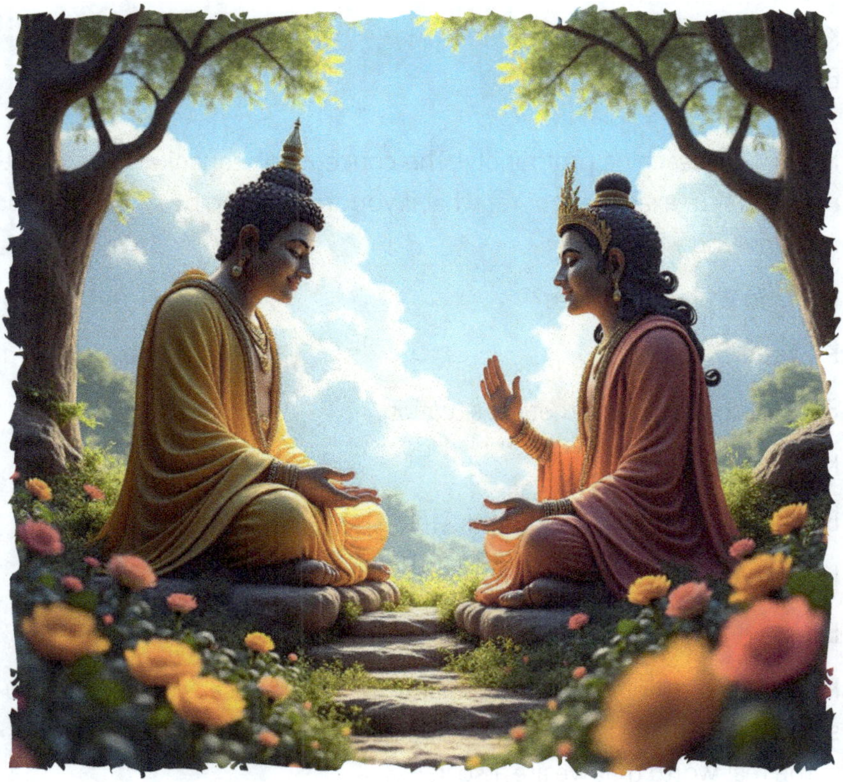

Bollytooth

The scene is a chaotic movie set in Bollywood (the film industry center in north Mumbai.)

The prevailing odor is a mix of hairspray and curry. The main set has a dramatic encounter between two of history's most illustrious personages, Krishna and the Buddha.

The set depicts a splendid forest, with an ancient mystical structure that appears to be a working temple, nestled in the foliage.

The scene unfolds:
Krishna actor = K
Buddha actor = B

K: "You are teaching profoundly! The concepts of equanimity, peacefulness and self-examination. Yet what if you are attacked by someone? You must defend yourself!"

B: "Who is being attacked?"

K: "Yourself."

B: "You express a hypothetical situation."

K: "Please, pretend it."

B: "I defend myself by being peaceful."

K: "But you shall be hurt this way."

B: "Again, a hypothetical situation."

K: "Excuse me, but we might benefit from hypothetical situations because then we can conjure up a solution in our imagination that might work in the real world that we are also in."

B: "Oh?"

K: "Thus, hypothetical situations may serve a useful purpose."

B: "Possibly."

K: "It's a dream world to be created so that when the real world comes, you are already prepared."

B: "I comprehend your reasoning. However, might this also apply to medicine where someone is given a mild poison in order to prepare them for a bigger poison?"

K: "Well, this is controversial, but it is the way of doing things. Zeus and Hades have confirmed this."

B: "Whom?"

K: "Oh, they are simply connected to the recycling business."

B: "You speak of deep things, Krishna."

K: "I'm sorry to bring this up."

B: "It's all right. May I then ask you something?"

K: "Please."

B: "I understand that you were a very happy-go-lucky yogi in the forest frolicking with the several gopis, the lovely maidens there."

K: "Yes, of course."

B: "And you would play tricks on them. You would steal their clothing while they were bathing in the river, and hide their clothing up in the trees."

K: "Oh, you recall it?"

B: "Therefore, they had to come out naked, and you could enjoy this frolicking with great, great pleasure and joy, watching them come out naked like this."

K: "Oh, it was sublime."

B: "And then you would take your flute and play it, and they would ask you, 'Why are you playing your flute here? We are naked. Why aren't you doing something more appropriate than playing your flute, you silly, silly yogi?'"

K: "Ah, yes. So legendary."

B: "And then you would say, 'Yes, but this is getting me prepared. This is the preparation phase for my next appropriate action, you see.' And they would reply, 'Ahh, that's very clever.'"

K: "I do love the gopis so very much."

B: "So they would ask you, 'Well, please give us our clothing back.' And you would say, 'No, no, no. I shall keep the clothing in the trees until you are ready to receive your clothing again.'"

K: "Oh, I agree, this was so clever."

B: "Yes. However, later on we see you in a war chariot, many years later, next to your disciple Arjuna.

We see you riding in the war chariot saying, 'Arjuna, you must fight this war and destroy all these enemies of yours. Even though they happen to be your own cousins, the children of your father's brother, or your mother's sister. They are your cousins, but you must destroy them.'"

K: "Oh, did you need to bring up the Gita here? I was so enjoying the gopi recollection."

B: "And why should you urge warlike destructions this way? For the record, you reasoned that it scarcely mattered, because they would all go to see God anyway. I have very deep questions about this, Krishna."

K: "Ah yes. I do also. I think this was a different Krishna. I'm just a happy yogi."

B: "Well, I need to know because you advocated much violence in that situation."

K: "Please let me explain. You are the Blessed One, who advocated for non-violence. This we know. You only know peacefulness. You only know tranquility. You only know peace of mind. You do this because the future is the result of the past."

B: "This is correct, Krishna. Your karmic trajectory steers your current path into your future circumstances."

K: "And so, if I want to enjoy a beautiful blissful future, I shall learn to be peaceful in this present existence, in this present moment?"

B: (nods) "Thus will you enjoy the follow-through of this karmic trajectory, which will bring you back to many great happy times again."

K: "You are so correct in this, O Blessed One! And by advocating violence rather than a peaceful solution, I might well find myself embroiled in countless wars into the future. Perhaps even as a victim."

B: "Of course, Krishna. And so you understand the karmic trajectory."

K: "Indeed, O Blessed One. May I become your disciple then?"

B: "Now?"

K: "Of course. Thus I shall return to being like the happy yogi I was before."

B: "This is so auspicious. And may I ask, what do you do in the real world, actor Krishna?"

K: "Oh, I'm an endodontist."

B: "No way!"

K: "The work is a bit slow, so I must act in order to boost my income."

B: "Ah, me also."

K: "Sure. Oops. I notice the director is waving furiously. We've gone very far off script. Not good."

B: "Actually he is rolling his arms. He bids us continue. I fancy he rather likes our improvisation."

K: "Let us nail it then!"

B: "Definitely. So you are an endo! I take it you perform root canal procedures?"

K: "Oh, so many that I've lost count!"

B: "This is not good."

K: "How so?"

B: "These are no longer living teeth. You might have saved them!"

K: "But how, good Sir? And may I ask, what is your stock in trade?"

B: "I'm actually a dental hygienist. I specialize in non-invasive treatments. Hence my current role."

K: "Oh, this is so serendipitous!"

B: "I fancy it is. But you need to use an ozone therapy along with pulp revitalization. Drill-free if possible."

K: "Oh, you understand it! I must speak to you at length about this! I have much to learn!"

B: "Of course. We shall go to a good café in Colaba and sip lattes, and I shall explain all the correct protocols."

K: "Oh, I feel like the happy yogi again! Oh wait, that was only the part I was playing…"

B: "But is it not all a play? Look, the director is coming over now."

K: "He wants to dismiss us?"

(*The director faces the actors and gives a big thumbs-up. He adjourns filming for the day, wearing a large smile.*)

B: "Let us be off then! I have much to tell you!"

K: "You do! Shall we stay in costume?"

B: "Of course. No need to change."

K: "But we shall draw crowds!"

B: "We are used to this!"

The ending of this film has dental students in sky-blue uniforms backflipping over dental chairs, as a hail of colorful confetti rains down.

70

CHAPTER

Return

Core points:

1. A large number of people avoid dentists altogether.
2. A.R.T. will be an ideal method to regain their trust.

There's a history of pitchfork-wielding gangs wanting to take out folks who "done them wrong".

Folks who cause damage, then charge AGAIN to fix what they did wrong! Not nice!

Better than pitchforks is to open a "solution clinic" instead.

The Luminara Dental Healing Spa is named after one of our amazing dentifrice brands (Chapter 55), and will specialize in ART treatments.

WE NEED A POSTER!

[We're here to welcome you back to happy, safe, and healing dental treatment.

We're the Luminara Dental Spa!

All right, you haven't been to a dentist in years. Why? Because, frankly, you're terrified!

We understand. That's why we launched Luminara!

We don't do synthetic smile marketing here. We're not into optics. We're about reality!

That reality is healing. We call it dental longevity.

Our foundation is drill-free treatment. Atraumatic and non-toxic. You'll enjoy your time here!

And you thought dentistry had to be terrifying. Have we got a surprise for you!

Find us at:

We're waiting for you. Your teeth have been neglected for years. That's wrong.

Come on over, and we'll show you how dental treatment was always supposed to be.]

There's our poster! We might add something along the bottom:

"They trade minutes in the chair for years of tooth lifespan - Claudio Pereira." We get it.

We hang this piece of brilliance in shopping malls and community centers. Places where folks who have suffered much, but now try to avoid pain, might congregate.

It's mostly these folks we're trying to reach. The Avoiders.

Soon, everyone will show up to our clinic, because that's how it goes when you offer folks what they actually need!

71

CHAPTER

RCT *Solutions*

Core points:

1. Root canal treatments carry risk.
2. They require regular monitoring.
3. Endodontics must become responsible and learn about ozone disinfection.

There has been serious concern over root canal treatments (RCTs). They are just too risky from a bacterial standpoint.

Dentists are persuasive, so many people have them. If you have one, the solution is to manage it.

There are basically two options: regular ozone treatment, or extraction.

Endodontists usually aren't interested in follow-up monitoring, but they need to be! In addition, most endodontists do not know about ozone! A radical problem!

They perform the RCTs but ignore checking the long-term effects of what they do! Another incredible footnote in dentistry.

I asked Nayera, a truth-seeking Cairo dentist, to provide a detailed position on root canals. She says:

1. "Dentinal tubules, millions of microscopic channels branching from the pulp chamber, remain beyond the reach of files and sealers. (This seems to be ignored in dental college.)
2. Intricate and porous, they may harbor bacteria that cannot be completely sterilized.
3. They risk being long-term reservoirs of toxins.

4. Obturation with latex or gutta-percha does not eliminate the bacterial threat, it merely encases it."

The good news:

1. "Ozone, in concentrated medical forms, penetrates dentin with a power that traditional irrigants lack.
2. The antimicrobial effect is rapid and expansive, disrupting bacterial membranes and neutralizing toxins.
3. It's used during the procedure and in regular recall visits.
4. It reduces bacterial load while preserving the natural structure of the tooth."

Finally:

1. "When infection proves resilient, extraction must be considered not as defeat but as a decisive act of healing.
2. Dentistry has too often been guided by tradition and economics rather than wellness."

Nayera adds: "To oppose RCTs is not to oppose dentistry. It is to reimagine it, to return to the root meaning of our duty: to reduce suffering, not cause it."

This analysis is remarkably lucid.

Anyone with RCTs must find good ozone therapy wherever available. The teeth are not attached to the jawbone for a reason. It's the Creator's wisdom. Extraction can actually be a solution to bacterial risk.

The correct Huggins protocol must always be followed. Mainly, that the periodontal ligament is removed as well.

Nearly all these RTCs might have been prevented in the first place! Actual proven tooth saving protocols are available!

But the knowledge was lacking! A much-too familiar refrain in the field of endodontics!

Healing capability in dentistry lacking? Whoa… Not possible!

72

CHAPTER

Undercover *Interview*

Core points:

1. Dentistry is a top-down hierarchy.
2. A healing approach is possible by active engagement.
3. A.R.T. could be the most valuable component of the dental curriculum.

I met a fully qualified dentist from a central Asian country whose degree wasn't recognized in Canada. He was applying to have it certified as a Canadian degree. Meantime, he worked as a receptionist in a local dental office.

I learned that he was fully trained in ART! I was very surprised. He agreed to answer a few questions. Here is a transcript:

C = coach (of dental healing)

D = dentist

C: You've had training in ART! Virtually no micro-fracturing or pulp trauma, plus stress-free!

D: Yes, but it's mostly done where they don't have access to dental drills. We did ART when we needed the tooth to hold over until we could do an RCT on it.

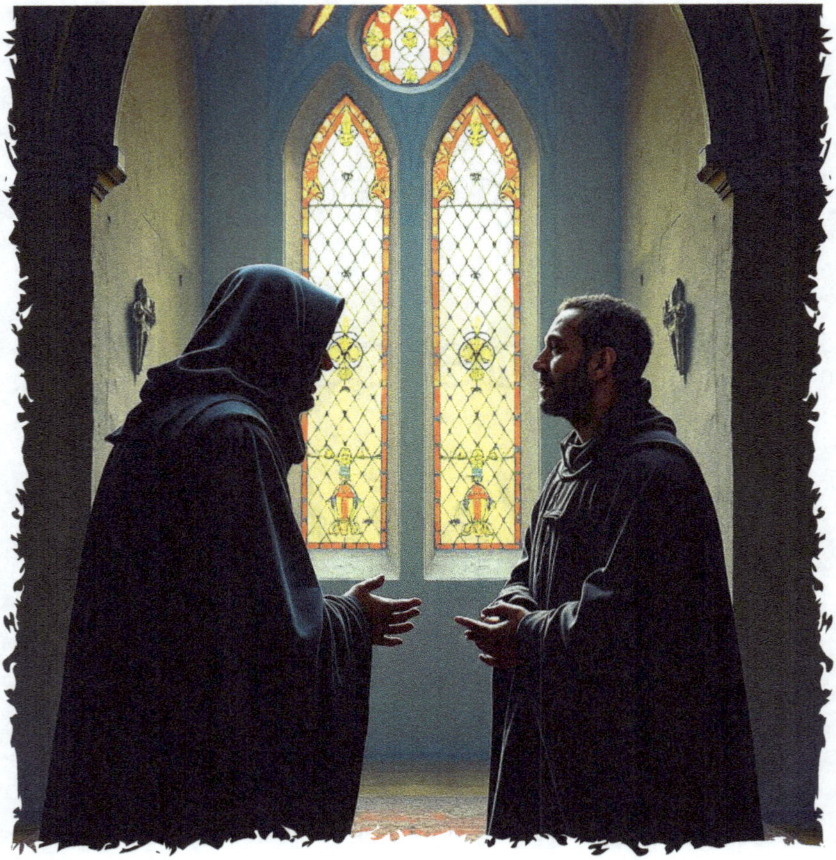

C: Seriously? It was only a patch until you could kill that tooth?

D: It's the standard of care.

C: Grrrrrrrr! Grrrrrrr! Grrrrrr!

D: Sorry….

C: Why was the ART filling only temporary?

D: It wasn't always. It can definitely last for years like any other filling, but if possible, it should be replaced by a regular composite.

C: Even if it's good and durable?

D: Hmmm. Maybe.

C: A 2007 study by Mickenautsch showed that ART restorations have superior longevity to drill fillings, with better seal quality.

D: Really?

C: If your prep is really good, you've removed all the soft decay but there's still discolored but firm dentin, do you leave it the way it is?

D: Dentin with the GIC could just turn to tertiary dentin, so we don't remove it. We try to preserve natural viable tooth structure.

C: That's the correct way. Do you know about Souza, a Brazilian researcher who did a lot of study on ART?

D: No.

C: Frencken?

D: No.

C: They're pioneers in ART. Who taught you the protocol?

D: It's something that's passed on. Whoever's teaching operative. I was actually teaching it myself by the end.

C: Were they full dentists?

D: They were dentists and specialists.

C: They learned the ART in the curriculum?

D: It's a newer part of the curriculum.

C: Many top quality studies prove that drilling causes micro-fracturing and pulp trauma.

D: Really?

C: Yes, Brännström, Elderton, and many others.

D: I never heard about these.

C: Do you question drilling in your own practice?

D: I'm not sure.

C: Pulp trauma is under 1% for ART, and over 60% for drill.

D: Really?

C: Restoration survival rates for ART are many times better.

D: That's new for me. But for a tooth with irreversible pulpitis, you'd need the drill.

C: You're talking about a root canal?

D: Yes.

C: Advanced pulpitis and even the necrotic tooth can still be saved with a combination of ART and aggressive ozone treatment.

D: You sure?

C: Yes. It's inexcusable that you were never taught about this. You paid serious money for that program too.

D: Yeah.

C: Should every tooth be saved if possible?

D: Yes, we should preserve as much tooth viable tooth structure as possible.

C: Do drills might take away viable dental structure?

D: They try to minimize damage to the tooth.

C: Have you ever had clients refuse drilling altogether and only accept an ART treatment?

D: No, I haven't.

C: Shouldn't they be lining up for it?

D: Looks like it.

C: If dentistry is stress-free, effective, relaxing, and also vastly healthier, then obviously it's preferable, right?

D: For sure.

C: Did your college discuss tooth longevity?

D: It got mentioned.

C: Would you do an ART restoration treatment as a freelancer?

D: I'm not allowed to.

C: By whom?

D: By the licensing boards.

C: Let's say someone had a car dealership and they didn't allow any other car dealerships, say, by having the mayor or the police stop them. Would that be a mafia?

D: Of course.

C: And if no one is allowed to do any other dentistry than the one standard method, and yet it's often injurious, what do you call that?

D: Can't really comment on that.

C: Thanks.

This interview took place in Vancouver BC, in May of 2025.

It wasn't sanctioned by any German philosophers...

73 CHAPTER

Ein Kaffeehaus 4

At a terrace cafe next to the Gera river in Erfurt, colorful flowerpots of bright pansies and chrysanthemums hang from railings. At a worn wooden table, three dentist-philosophers, Dr. Georg Hegel, Dr. Karl Jaspers, and Dr. Martin Heidegger, are now joined by theologians Martin Luther and Meister Eckhart. The waiter brings two more cups of hot latte.

Luther: "Gentlemen, you called Herr Eckhart and me over to your table because you are troubled in your practice!"

Hegel: "It's true. We cannot continue as secret dentists. It's unsustainable."

Jaspers: "People are whispering!"

Heidegger: "The dental boards are becoming suspicious. All our clients are receiving excellent healing results, with minimal pain and discomfort!"

Eckhart: "Then it's radical! You have arrived at Gelassenheit, the releasement from harmful method!"

Jaspers: "But now we have to give up philosophy. It's a tenuous limit-situation!"

Hegel: "Why give it up? A healing method is simply a higher philosophy."

Heidegger: "But our logical frameworks ... our academic tenure..."

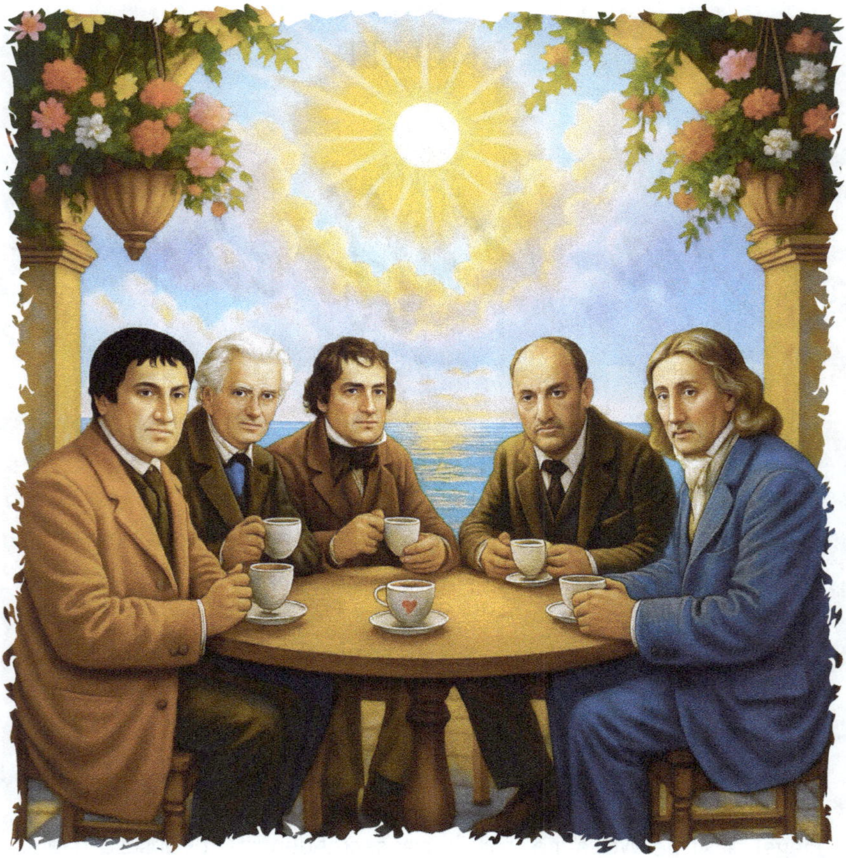

Luther: "There is only one framework, and that is the Radiant Truth! It goes far beyond rational principles. However, it requires official excommunication as a rite of passage! Nasty discomfort!"

Eckhart: "Herr Luther studied my experience. He keeps this a secret. Gentlemen, you must become excommunicated from the rigid corporate limitations! You must embrace this rite of passage! It is rebirth!"

Japers: "Ahh, invasive corporate dentistry forcing us into a cathartic, phoenix-like transformation!"

Heidegger: "I like this very much!"

Hegel: "I do also. It seems to be the synthesis of the dentistry-healing thesis-antithesis."

Luther: (*stands abruptly*) "Nein! There is more! There is the unfound passion, seeking to be discovered!"

Jaspers: "I now tremble."

Eckhart: "Herr Martin must stand when excited. He has low tolerance for dry logic."

Luther: "The atraumatic method must prevail, just as the Holy One prevailed in the dialogue of truth!"

Hegel: "Prevailed and proceeded! I'm a secret Murshid."

Jaspers: "A Persian mystic?"

Hegel: "I don't advertise."

Heidegger: "Then it's all logical now! My Daesin described only a fraction of the possible states of being! The Three Suns! Imagine it!"

Eckhart: "Relax. We grow from children to adulthood."

Jaspers: "Then our dentistry must also grow up! It must become the craft it's truly meant to be!"

Eckhart: "Of course, gentlemen."

Hegel: "Horcht! There is a new brauhaus down the way! It serves the finest pilsners from the Bohemian forest lands!"

Luther: "Then why do we delay?" (*Grabs both Jaspers and Heidegger by the collar and pulls them up.*)

Eckhart: (*to Hegel*) "You must tell me all about this new ART protocol!"

Hegel: "Ich werde! I shall!"

74

CHAPTER

True Dentistry

The full case has been made.

Painful, traumatic, stressful dentistry is in a majority of cases completely unnecessary.

Gentle, easy-going, enjoyable dentistry is not only possible, but it's also far healthier for you.

Sure, it's a sea change. It turns the whole game upside down.

This approach saves needless suffering and pain for countless numbers of people; for everyone that ever goes to a regular dentist.

Definitely a good deal. When you find good deals, you take them. You don't ask a lot of questions.

This stylistic approach involved using drama, humor, and parody to make the topic relatable and understandable for a broad audience, not just experts.

The goal was to demonstrate that this improved dental experience is achievable, accessible, and not complicated. It is highly desirable, necessary, and long overdue.

Website: dentalhealer.com
dentalhealer@yandex.com

ABOUT THE AUTHOR:

Oba is Robert Godbout's secret nickname.
Three letter elegance, compared to thirteen
The Golden Sun, radiant and aflame,
A dental longevity concept so keen.
Biographies look to the past at what's already been.

Upstream, a challenging directional place.
The light that's to come, a majestic allure.
A splendor of potency in a magical space,
Brilliant realms blaze all the cares into cures,
Shining the vindication of truth, eternally pure.

Oba wanders a planet without fail,
Golden orbs indicating the way to and fro.
Then a Salish Sea return to pick up the mail.
Comedy routines once performed long ago.
Light Wizards of wisdom point out a new glow.

AFTER-NOTES AND CITATIONS OF STUDIES:

1. **Arvit Banerjee (2000):** Arvit Banerjee and R. J. Elderton, "The Need for Rethinking the Use of Rotary Cutting Instruments," Dental Update 27, no. 4 (May 2000): 186-192.

2. **Brännström (1965):** Martin Brännström and Göran Johnson, "Effects of Various Conditioners and Cleaning Agents on Prepared Dentin Surfaces: A Scanning Electron Microscopic Investigation," Journal of Prosthetic Dentistry 31, no. 4 (April 1974): 422-430. (Note: The seminal 1965 study is often cited in texts but is a conference proceeding. The 1974 paper is the key, widely accessible journal article on the same topic by Brännström).

3. **Elderton study:** R. J. Elderton, "The Causes of Failure of Restorations: A Literature Review," Journal of Dentistry 4, no. 6 (December 1976): 257-262. (This is a classic review on iatrogenic damage from drilling, among other causes).

4. **Pereira study:** Cláudio Pereira, "Atraumatic Restorative Treatment (ART) for Dental Caries," Journal of the Indian Society of Pedodontics and Preventive Dentistry 14, no. 1 (March 1996): 1-4.

5. **Frencken study on ART efficacy:** Jo E. Frencken et al., "Effectiveness of ART and Traditional Amalgam Restorations in Permanent Teeth: A Meta-analysis," Journal of Dental Research 91, no. 10 (October 2012): 914-920, https://doi.org/10.1177/0022034512458687.

6. **Souza (Brazil) public health ART study:** M. S. Souza et al., "Two-Years Survival Rate of Atraumatic Restorative Treatment (ART) and Sealants in a School-Based Oral Health Programme in Piracicaba, SP, Brazil," Journal of Applied Oral Science 21, no. 3 (June 2013): 224-230, https://doi.org/10.1590/1679-775720130064.

7. **Fusayama study on dental drill harm:** Takao Fusayama and Masashi Ide, "The Surface of Mechanically Exposed Dentin," Bulletin of the Tokyo Medical and Dental University 10, no. 2 (June 1963): 135-148.

CLARIFICATIONS AND CONTEXT:

Arvit Banerjee (2000): This is a co-authored paper with Professor Elderton. It is a review and opinion piece arguing for a more conservative, minimally invasive approach to cavity preparation, directly addressing the harm caused by traditional drilling.

Brännström (1965): The 1965 reference is to Martin Brännström's theory of "dentinal sensitivity," first fully articulated in his book Dentinal and Pulpal Response (1965). The 1974 paper is the classic experimental work that provided the visual evidence (via SEM) for the "smear layer" and its effects.

Elderton Study: Professor R. John Elderton was a prolific researcher on the reasons for restoration failure. His 1976 review is a foundational text identifying how cavity preparation itself (i.e., the drill) is a primary cause of future problems.

Pereira Study: This citation is for a key early paper by Dr. Cláudio Pereira, a Brazilian dentist who was instrumental in the early research and promotion of ART alongside Jo Frencken and others.

Frencken Study: Professor Jo Frencken is one of the principal inventors of the ART technique. This 2012 meta-analysis is a major, high-impact study demonstrating the long-term efficacy of ART in permanent teeth, making it a landmark citation.

Souza (Brazil) Study: This is an example of a real-world public health implementation study of ART in a Brazilian school program, demonstrating its practicality and success in a non-clinical setting.

Fusayama Study: This is the seminal early work by Takao Fusayama distinguishing between the infected and affected dentin layers. His research showed that complete removal of all discolored dentin (often done with a drill) was unnecessary and harmful to the tooth structure.

ADDITIONAL REFERENCES:

8. **James H. Zach and Stanley Cohen, "Thermogenesis in Operative Techniques:** Comparison of Four Methods," Journal of Prosthetic Dentistry 12, no. 5 (September–October 1962): 977-984. https://doi.org/10.1016/0022-3913(62)90183-3.

9. **Mickenautsch:** Steffen Mickenautsch is a leading researcher in systematic reviews of ART. A key citation is: Steffen Mickenautsch, V. C. C. Marinho, and S. R. Yengopal, "Caries-Preventive Effect of High-Viscosity Glass Ionomer and Resin-Based Fissure Sealants on Permanent Teeth: A Systematic Review of Clinical Trials," PLOS ONE 11, no. 1 (January 2016): e0146512. https://doi.org/10.1371/journal.pone.0146512.

10. **Pashley (Smear Layer & Dentin Permeability):** David H. Pashley, "Smear Layer: Physiological Considerations," Operative Dentistry 9, suppl. 3 (1984): 13-29.

11. **Langeland (Pulp Response to Trauma):** Kaare Langeland, "Tissue Response to Dental Caries," Endodontics & Dental Traumatology 3, no. 4 (August 1987): 149-171. https://doi.org/10.1111/j.1600-9657.1987.tb00619.x.

12. **Ericson (Cavity Preparation & Bacterial Leakage):** Dan Ericson, Martin Brännström, and K. Nordenvall, "Contamination of Dentin Surfaces with Vital and Devitalized Bacteria: Effect on Diffusion of Bacteria through Dentin," Swedish Dental Journal 9, no. 5 (1985): 185-192.

13. **Stanley (Pulp Biology & Injury):** Harold R. Stanley, "Design for a Human Pulp Study Part II," Oral Surgery, Oral Medicine, Oral Pathology 25, no. 5 (May 1968): 756-764. https://doi.org/10.1016/0030-4220(68)90024-0.

CLARIFICATIONS AND CONTEXT:

Zach & Cohen (1962): This is arguably the most important study ever published on the danger of thermal trauma from drilling. It was scientifically established that a temperature rise of 5.5°C (10°F) above normal is the critical threshold beyond which irreversible pulpitis and necrosis occur. This paper is the reason modern dentistry mandates water coolant and controlled handpiece speed.

Mickenautsch: The work provides high-level evidence (via systematic reviews and meta-analyses) that minimally invasive techniques like ART are not just alternatives but are often superior in terms of long-term outcomes and pulp health compared to traditional drill-and-fill, especially in certain clinical situations.

Pashley (1984): This paper is a comprehensive review of the "smear layer" – the layer of debris created by the drill that clogs dentinal tubules. It discusses how this layer affects permeability, bonding, and bacterial leakage, which are central to the concepts of pulpal harm and restoration failure.

Langeland (1987): A classic review from a pioneering oral pathologist detailing the biological response of the dental pulp to various insults, including the mechanical trauma of cavity preparation, thermal injury, and bacterial microleakage.

Stanley (1968): Part of a series of famous human pulp studies that meticulously documented the inflammatory response of the human dental pulp to different operative procedures and materials, providing a biological basis for minimally invasive dentistry.

75

BONUS CHAPTER

Safe *Removals*

If you have mercury amalgam fillings, and choose to remove them, you'll be lifting a serious source of toxicity from your system.

This is not advice, it's just evidence. That's why we need the disclaimer:

[Disclaimer: This information is for educational purposes only and is not medical advice. The choice of removal technique is a personal one that must be made in consultation with a qualified dental professional. Discuss the risks, benefits, and alternatives thoroughly with your dental healer.]

A 4-POINT MODULE ON AMALGAM REMOVAL STYLES & SAFETY:

Point 1: The Conventional Removal

Description: This involves a high-speed drill (handpiece) with significant water coolant and high-volume suction. The goal is to section the amalgam and remove it efficiently, often under a rubber dam for isolation.

Backers: It's the technique taught in dental schools worldwide, coming soon after the poison class on how to place this mercury amalgam.

Ship of fools, anyone? The major dental associations and boards go this route.

Safety Protocols: Use of rubber dam, high-volume suction, water coolant to minimize heat and aerosol.

Success Probability for Minimal Harm: Very High (>95%).

Point 2: The "Biological / Holistic" Approach

Description: Minimizes patient exposure to amalgam particles and vapor during removal. Employs a more stringent set of safety protocols.

Backers: Organizations like the International Academy of Oral Medicine and Toxicology (IAOMT). Goal is to reduce all potential risk from mercury exposure.

Safety Protocols: The "SMART" (Safe Mercury Amalgam Removal Technique) protocol includes: supplemental oxygen for the patient, a rubber dam, high-volume suction outside the dam, specialized vacuum air filters, and chunking the amalgam to reduce drilling.

Success Probability for Minimal Harm: High (~90-95%).

Point 3: The Huggins Protocol (Allergy/Toxicity Focus)

Description: It says that amalgam removal can trigger immune and detoxification responses and must be done in a specific sequence alongside nutritional support.

Key Sources & Philosophy: Devised by long-term dental mercury opponent Hal Huggins. Addresses the range of mercury-related autoimmune and chronic illnesses; removal must be managed to avoid "detox crises."

Safety Protocols: Similar to IAOMT (rubber dam, suction) but with galvanic and compatibility testing for replacement materials, and pre- and post-treatment nutritional regimens.

Success Probability for Minimal Harm: Lack of industry-led testing and measures.

Point 4: The Hand-Instrument Only Method

Description: Using only spoon excavators, hatchets, and other non-rotary instruments to pry and scrape the amalgam out.

Key Sources & Philosophy: Often requested by patients with extreme fear of drills or belief that vibration causes more toxicity.

Safety Protocols: Rubber dam is absolutely mandatory. The process is slow and methodical.

Success Probability for Minimal Harm: Low to Moderate (<70%).

Contains a risk of tooth fracture and the difficulty of complete removal. This is because it requires a physical force to break up the metal amalgam.

These are the main choices, and any decision should be made in close collaboration with very qualified and healing-minded professionals.

The rubber dam is a key feature of all these protocols. It's a latex-nitrite sheet that isolates the tooth being worked on from the rest of the mouth. It's an absolute must.

Suction and air filtration are equally essential. They significantly reduce the amount of aerosol and vapor the patient and staff are exposed to.

Water coolant is a must in any drilling treatment, despite that it doesn't fully reach the contact point. However, it does reduce the amount of mercury vapor released during drilling by over 90%.

The "Chunking vs. Grinding" debate:

"Chunking" involves using a drill to cut the amalgam into large segments that can be lifted out, minimizing the grinding of the amalgam into a fine powder. It's a common-sense technique that is effective and reduces potential exposure.

Summary of methods:

The hand-instrument only (ART-style) method is rated at only 70% risk-free due to the risk of mechanical damage to the tooth structure. The skill of the practitioner is paramount.

The IAOMT SMART protocol probably represents the most cautious, technologically advanced approach for those deeply concerned about mercury exposure.

The Huggins protocol involves extra detox methods that need to be well evaluated.

Mark Breiner is a dentist with a book "Whole Body Dentistry".

He recounts two first-hand experiences with mercury toxicity:

1. "A patient of mine told me about the terrible health problems her young son was encountering. He would get so sick every few weeks that he would be unable to walk and had to be hospitalized. The doctors at the medical centre were able to confirm that there was something wrong with his immune system, but they did not know what was causing the problem. I asked my patient if any dental work had recently been done on the child. Sure enough a Pedodontist had placed amalgams and stainless steel (nickel) crowns in his mouth. I explained my suspicions to her, and she brought the child in right away. After I removed the metals from his mouth, the child recovered immediately. In the many years since this happened, he has never had a recurrence of his original problem."

2. "When Tiffany was three, her Pedodontist recommended and placed amalgam fillings and stainless steel crowns in her mouth. Immediately following the procedure, this previously healthy, active toddler became ill and had a dramatic increase in her white cell count. For a full year, she did not gain a pound, suffered from recurrent fevers, low energy, and a diminished immune system. When she finally came to me, I recommended that she be tested, immunologically, for dental materials. She was found to be reactive to both mercury and nickel. We removed all the metals in her mouth, and she is now fine. The severe illness was simply a normal physical reaction to being poisoned by metals that the small child's system simply could not handle."

These stories are actually commonplace. They come under the heading: Dental Iatrogenesis.

May you never have to experience this. May your teeth be fit, well, and trouble-free.

May you know what's good for your teeth and how to avoid harmful treatments. Then, you can focus on the super-happiest things!

Notes

Notes

Notes

Notes

Notes

Notes

Notes

Notes

Notes

www.ingramcontent.com/pod-product-compliance
Lightning Source LLC
LaVergne TN
LVHW010713061126
851857LV00014B/1167